A Natural Approach

ALLERGIES

Macrobiotic Health Education Series

MACROBIOTIC HEALTH EDUCATION SERIES

A Natural Approach

ALLERGIES

by Michio Kushi

edited by Mark Mead and John David Mann

foreword by Marc Van Cauwenberghe, M.D.

JP

Japan Publications, Inc.

Tokyo • New York

Illustrations by Rosalind Rhodes

Note to the reader: Those with health problems are advised to seek the guidance of a qualified medical, or psychological professional in addition to that of a qualified macrobiotic counselor before implementing any of the dietary and other approaches presented in this book. It is essential that any reader who has any reason to suspect serious illness in themselves or their family members seek appropriate medical, nutritional, or psychological advice promptly. Neither this or any other health related book should be used as a substitute for qualified care or treatment.

Published by JAPAN PUBLICATIONS, INC., Tokyo and New York

Distributors:
UNITED STATES: *Kodansha International/USA, Ltd., through Harper & Row, Publishers, Inc., 10 East 53rd Street, New York, New York 10022.* SOUTH AMERICA: *Harper & Row, Publishers, Inc., International Department.* CANADA: *Fitzhenry & Whiteside Ltd., 195 Allstate Parkway, Markham, Ontario, L3R 4T8.* MEXICO AND CENTRAL AMERICA: *HARLA S. A. de C. V., Apartado 30–546, Mexico 4, D. F.* BRITISH ISLES: *International Book Distributors Ltd., 66 Wood Lane End, Hemel Hempstead, Herts HP2 4RG.* EUROPEAN CONTINENT: *Fleetbooks, S. A., c/o Feffer and Simons (Nederland) B. V., Rijnkade 170, 1382 GT Weesp, The Netherlands.* AUSTRALIA AND NEW ZEALAND: *Bookwise International, 1 Jeanes Street, Beverley, South Australia 5007.* THE FAR EAST AND JAPAN: *Japan Publications Trading Co., Ltd., 1–2–1, Sarugaku-cho, Chiyoda-ku, Tokyo 101.*

First edition: May 1985

LCCC No. 84–081354
ISBN 0–87040–616–7

Printed in U.S.A.

Foreword

For the past 12 years I have been offering macrobiotic advice for many health problems. Although I obtained a medical degree several years before that, I myself was not a healthy person. I suffered from several skin problems (*furunculosis* was one of them), allergies (*hives*), intestinal problems and emotional disturbances, and I couldn't cure or even improve any of them. Through my training as a doctor I received very little awareness of the existence of any relationship between food, blood, and health. And although I knew that, medically speaking, chocolate was not helpful in cases of furunculosis, I couldn't stop eating it, because it was a source of happiness for me.

I did not enjoy working as a general practitioner. Although patients were praising me, I did not get any deep satisfaction out of my work. I had not learned to deal with health problems except with injections or by prescribing drugs, and I noticed that not infrequently I created new problems by doing this. I made a good income, but felt like a slave. I relieved symptoms, but felt like a drug dealer.

For almost two years I then worked as a coroner, wanting to become a pathologist. Practically every day I autopsied whoever had died in the hospital, trying to discover the cause of death. Again I witnessed how mankind is suffering, how little modern medicine can do, and how often it makes mistakes. Simultaneously, I took care of my mother who was dying of metastasized breast cancer. In the course of a year I saw a strong optimistic woman change into a chronically tortured, desperate living skeleton, although she received all possible medical care, and she kept eating a strengthening diet.

Surrounded by sickness, despair and death I stumbled upon a book by George Ohsawa, *Cancer and the Philosophy of the Far East*, which turned out to contain the secret of health, happiness and life. I didn't understand too much of the book, and I thought it was rather philosophical, but it fascinated me and contained some practical guidelines. Purely out of curiosity I started to try them, and to my surprise, within weeks, all of my former health troubles started to vanish, one by one. Without hesitation I then quit my job and devoted years to the study of macrobiotics, because I was fortunate enough to find out about Mr. Michio Kushi. He turned out to be much more fascinating than any of the hundred professors I studied with.

I can understand the criticism or scepticism that many scientists and doctors have about macrobiotics. Their method of acquiring knowledge cannot allow any acknowledgment without hard evidence. We can only invite them to practice the macrobiotic way of living for several months. In this way they will have a basis upon which to judge its effects. I extend this same invitation to you. After all, "seeing is believing."

MARC VAN CAUWENBERGHE, M.D.
Brookline, Massachusetts
November, 1984

Introduction

Our purpose in presenting the *Macrobiotic Health Education Series* is two-fold. The primary concern, of course, has been to present the reader with the practical application of macrobiotic principles, through daily eating and lifestyle, to a broad range of specific health problems. In contrast to the modern trend towards specialization, the macrobiotic approach to health aims at nourishing and restoring the whole person to a naturally healthy, happy condition on all levels, including physical, emotional, mental and spiritual well-being. Because of this holistic scope, the practice of macrobiotics is naturally applicable to the widest range of different health problems. Macrobiotics, indeed, can be adapted to help alleviate virtually any aspect of human suffering, provided that appropriate modifications for each individual illness or circumstance are introduced with the proper understanding.

At the same time, the ancient unifying principle of yin and yang can be applied as a practical approach to studying and clarifying the various scientific riddles in a problem such as allergies, and offers a clear understanding of the origin, cause and mechanism of each problem under study.

On a broader level, each particular problem addressed in the *Health Education Series* also illustrates larger issues underlying our modern civilization's orientation, way of thinking and approach to life. By examining such philosophical questions, the *Health Education Series* is also presenting the larger goal of macrobiotics, which is to establish health at the individual, family and community levels as a first step towards solving larger social and national problems and, eventually, helping to create a firm foundation for health, happiness and peace on a global scale.

The central philosophical issue underlying the problem of allergies is that the precepts upon which our modern view of life is based are often those of defensiveness and a sense of separation from the natural world. The notion of the immune system battling against hostile elements in our surroundings—rather than as a natural mechanism for harmonizing our condition with the environment—is one example of an underlying view of separateness. We must ask ourselves if allergies are truly caused by things such as grasses, cats and dogs, wheat or beans, or even hot and cold temperatures, or if they are simply the result of our own internal imbalance. Is the flaw a part of nature, or in our own inability to adapt to nature?

Through macrobiotics, we are able to reunite with our surroundings. Practically speaking, by changing our biological condition through proper diet and lifestyle, we can successfully adapt and become an integral part of our environment, rather than a separate existence under siege. As thousands of people have experienced, allergic problems can improve with time and the proper attention and guidance. More broadly speaking, the application of macrobiotic principles to the problem of allergies can illustrate that we may find an effective, inexpensive and inherently peaceful solution to all antagonisms, real and imaginary.

The few anecdotal case histories presented in this volume represent only a sampling of the many such cases of improvement and recovery through macrobiotics we have witnessed over the past 30 years since macrobiotics has been introduced and developed in the Western world. During this time, the development of the macrobiotic movement has grown to encompass a broad range of educational activities, including a network of several hundred educational centers throughout the United States, Canada, Western Europe, South America and the Far East, as well as in parts of Eastern Europe, Africa, Australia and other countries. In the U.S. alone, over 15,000 natural foods, health foods and other stores now carry macrobiotic staple food supplies and literature on the macrobiotic approach to health. The basic tenets of the macrobiotic health approach have also begun to appear in major health agencies' research reports, such as the 1977 U.S. Senate report *Dietary Goals for the United States* and the 1982 National Research Council's report on *Diet, Nutrition and Cancer.* More recently, many medical doctors and scientific agencies have begun to work in collaboration with macrobiotic organizations such as the East West Foundation on research projects to document scientifically the efficacy of the macrobiotic approach in relieving illness.

We would like to thank all of the people who have contributed to these first volumes of the *Health Education Series.* We thank Iwao Yoshizaki, President of Japan Publications, Inc., and Yoshiro Fujiwara, the Japan Publications representative for America, for their guidance and advice, together with our macrobiotic associate Edward Esko. We also thank Phillip Janetta in Tokyo for editing the final text, and Rosalind Rhodes for providing the illustrations. Our gratitude also goes to Marc Van Cauwenberghe, M.D., for contributing the Foreword, and to all of our friends who wrote case histories. We also thank Aveline Kushi, Rosalind Rhodes, Olivia Oredson and Wendy Esko for their efforts in developing the companion volume in the *Macrobiotic Food and Cooking Series, Cooking for Health: Allergies.*

Allergies currently stand as one of our leading detriments to health. If we can change this difficulty into our benefactor and solve the problem of allergies through natural, peaceful means, then we are one step closer to our long-cherished dream of world health and world peace.

MICHIO KUSHI
MARK MEAD
JOHN DAVID MANN

Brookline, Massachusetts
November 1984

Contents

4. The Macrobiotic Approach to Allergies, 81

5. Approaching Individual Allergies, 101

6. Personal Experiences, 129

1. The Benign Environment

Allergy is one of the most common ailments of the modern world. It is estimated that at least one half of the entire world population suffers from some type of mild or serious allergy. In the United States, the prevalence of allergy has shown a steady increase over the last few decades. The 1967 medical statistics found an estimated 20 million people with allergies, with at least 50% of the American population exhibiting minor allergic tendencies at the time. By 1983, this number had nearly doubled to 39 million persons, or one out of every six Americans. Out of this 39 million, the allergic form of asthma afflicts 9 million people; over 18 million have hay fever alone, and the remaining 12 million are affected by other allergies. One should also realize that the 39 million figure is a conservative estimate, since many allergic cases either are not reported or go unrecognized in clinical diagnosis. Hay fever, for instance, is so common that most people choose to handle it on their own—by avoiding pollen-rich areas, staying indoors, carrying nasal decongestants, and so forth. As another example, food or chemical allergy is often either misdiagnosed or unsuspected, and some allergy specialists believe that this form alone affects well over 20 million people. One third of all chronic diseases in children under age seventeen are caused by asthma, hay fever, or other allergies, which makes allergy the most common form of disability among school children. Allergy is indeed so widespread that some medical doctors have estimated that 100 million Americans are hypersensitive, whether they know it or not.

Allergy not only constitutes a relentless bother throughout one's life, but may also result in unnatural death; asthma, for example, kills thousands of Americans each year. Another chronic respiratory condition, emphysema involves hardening of the lung tissue and the accumulation of fluids that choke off the oxygen supply to the blood, causing prolonged labored breathing and fatigue, ultimately leading to disability. Since the 1950's, the number of Americans dying from emphysema has risen almost logarithmically. Food allergy is now also suspected to underlie some cases of major illnesses, including hypoglycemia, arthritis, stroke, heart disease, and various cancers. A recent report stated that food allergy occurs in 15% of the adults and 40% of the children who have allergy symptoms of any kind. Among infants under two years of age, about 100% of all allergies are food allergies.

The problem becomes more disturbing when we consider recent medical surveys of school children and adult groups in areas ranging from Chicago to Denver to Montreal. In these studies, teams of doctors tested groups of unsuspecting, seemingly normal individuals for allergic reactions. They found that between 23% and 29% of those tested—an average of one in four—had allergies that could be diagnosed medically. Thus, it appears that many people are allergic but simply do not know it. In fact, the prestigious Allergy Foundation of America has stated that ". . . allergies may constitute one of the most widespread, undiagnosed diseases in the United States."

The Cost of Allergies

Undergoing conventional allergy treatment can be an expensive proposition, and these days fewer people are able to afford medical treatments for serious allergies. A complete allergy consultation with skin tests may cost over $400.00. Most professional consulations for allergy evaluation include a detailed history and physical examination, the cost of which may vary from $50 to $200. Skin testing alone often costs around $200. According to the popular book, *The Best Guide to Allergy*, desensitization shots during the first year could run anywhere from $400 to $1,250. Additional fees for supplemental diagnostic tests will further fatten the bill. Altogether, allergic people spend an estimated $250 million for medicines and another $200 million for injections annually. Furthermore, allergic patients require an average of three times as many medical visits as those with other types of illness.

Allergy treatments may be costly in other ways as well. For the large number of allergic Americans, there are relatively few allergists available, and still fewer certified by the Allergy Foundation of America or by the American Medical Association. It is also difficult to find a competent allergist, since many of these specialists have not kept pace with the more recent findings in immunology and the related areas of genetics and nutrition; also, very little training concerning the prevention and treatment of allergies is given either in medical school or during internship.

The biggest cost of allergies is to the individual. The most popular approach involves administering a series of allergy shots over a minimum of three years, or else an array of strong pharmaceutical drugs to eliminate symptoms, and these therapies often have dramatic side-effects on individual health. Other current approaches call for complex diets lacking variety or balanced nutritional quality; or, in more serious cases, for placing the individual in a sterile environment which severely restricts free movement or exploration. Allergic children must learn to avoid the kind of environment which might trigger an allergic reaction and thus do not grow up with the same pleasures enjoyed by other children in their age group. In-short, the greatest cost of allergy, as in all forms of illness, is the loss of individual freedom.

Limitations of the Microscopic View

The primary reason for the increasing incidence of allergy is that most people do not know the root cause of the disorder. Most medical authorities maintain that the more pertinent cause of allergy is the substance which triggers the allergic reaction—the so-called *allergen.* According to this view, the cause of hay fever is pollen; the cause of food allergy is the offending food; the cause of asthma is dust or some other particular environmental condition which elicits the asthmatic reaction; and the cause of direct-contact skin allergies is whatever the skin happens to be exposed to prior to the inflammatory response. The conventional approach is therefore based on the assumption that the allergen itself is, practically speaking, the main problem. Accordingly, the allergic person must first learn to avoid the allergen by whatever means possible. He or she may also be advised to take drugs which interfere with the microscopic allergic reaction, or with the development of symptoms associated with this reaction.

However, this view prompts the question: if the true cause of allergy is the allergen itself, then why isn't everyone allergic? With the recent surge of medical interest in allergic *susceptibility*, the latest approach has been to attribute allergic disorders to genetic abnormalities, since allergies often tend to "run in the family." Some scientists believe that it is the genetically tuned production of antibodies which determines allergic tendencies. To date, no clear genetic mechanism has been identified or established, and there are considerable inconsistencies with this answer. However, even if a clear genetic basis for allergic susceptibility were discovered, this would merely elicit the same question in another form: why should this genetic defect exist in only certain individuals, and why should it develop into full-blown allergy in one genetically prone person, yet not in another?

There are two basic flaws in the modern scientific line of inquiry, which have so far limited this approach to the extent that no satisfactory explanation or practical, lasting solution for the problem of allergy has been found. First, most conventional approaches are *microscopic* rather than *macroscopic*; they generally attempt to solve the problem on the mechanistic, cellular level, rather than beginning with a larger view of the fundamental relationship between human beings and the natural environment that creates, nourishes and sustains us. And second, if we do look from this larger perspective, we can see that the modern approach is intrinsically *dualistic*; that is, it is oriented by a viewpoint that sees human beings as separate existences within an essentially threatening environment, as represented in the common romantic image of "man battling the elements."

Dualism means that we see every problem in antagonistic terms, as friend and foe, good and bad, or invader and defender. Consequently, many health problems, including allergy, are viewed as instances of the body being unable to effectively "defend" against foreign, "hostile" invaders—in this case the offending allergens. The inevitable response is that of counterattack, which has led to the awesome arsenal of modern medical weaponry, from antibiotics and antihistamines to laser surgery, radiation therapy and chemotherapy. The annually increasing incidence of allergy in this country is only one example of the escalating spiral of hostilities this approach has produced.

The Macrobiotic Approach

The macrobiotic approach begins with the realization that the environment itself is orderly and supportive; and further, that human life is a natural, integral part of this constantly changing, harmonious fabric. When a problem arises, such as allergy, it is not that we are unable to defend properly against a foreign invader, but that we have made ourselves unable to respond appropriately and harmonize peacefully with our benign environment.

Under conditions of normal health, we are in a state of constant exchange with the world around us, through the absorption and elimination of solid matter, liquid, gasses, heat and various wavelengths of electromagnetic radiation. In the case of allergies, this exchange has become disorderly and chaotic; and the most basic source of this disorder is a long-term lack of natural order in our daily way of eating. The importance of properly managing our daily food becomes clear when we realize that the food and drink we take in every day constitutes our most fundamental cellular link with the natural world within which we live. Harmony within our own daily dietary practice, therefore, is the cornerstone of all traditional approaches to health, which have sought to maintain the natural, normal harmony between humanity and the universe. This traditional viewpoint is the cornerstone of the macrobiotic approach.

As both a philosophy and a way of life, macrobiotics was historically recognized in ancient Greece and in the Far East. The Greek term was *macrobios* which translates into "great life." In its more modern usage, macrobiotics has come to mean a way of life according to the largest possible view. The ancient Chinese considered macrobiotics to be the art of life and longevity, as the acclaimed historian Joseph Needham explained in his monumental work *Science and Civilization in China*. This seemingly abstract cosmology was based on a profound understanding of the natural laws of change and was incorporated into all aspects of daily life. The practice of macrobiotics involves understanding and applying this universal order of change to our lifestyle, including the selection, preparation, and manner of eating our daily food.

The Order of the Universe

By observing our day-to-day thoughts and activities, we can readily see that nothing in this universe is static or unchanging. Electrons move constantly around the central nucleus of the atom; the earth rotates on its axis while orbiting the sun; the solar system is revolving around the galaxy; and galaxies are moving away from each other with tremendous velocity, as the entire universe continues to expand. Within this unceasing movement, an order or pattern may be perceived. The light of day turns slowly into the dark of night, and then returns to day again. Winter changes gradually to summer and then back to winter again. During the day we stand up and are active, while at night we lie down and rest, or pursue more passive activities such as watching the movies. We begin human life as a single fertilized cell which grows into an embryo, then follow the processes of birth, growth, maturity, and death. These cycles of change occur throughout nature, and likewise influence all domains of human life.

Taking these common sense observations a step further, we see that change occurs according to certain natural laws or principles. The universal principle of all processes of change is the dialectical relationship of complementary opposites—or yin and yang. All phenomena are governed by the interplay of outward and inward movements or tendencies. Yin, or outward movement, results in expansion while yang, or inward movement, produces contraction. We observe these universal tendencies in the human body, for example, as the alternating expansion and contraction of the heart and lungs, or in the movements of the stomach and intestines during digestion. Temperature-wise, compression (yang) produces heat which eventually turns back to expansion (yin); while expansion produces coldness which then results in compression. In the winter our bodies contract to conserve heat. During the hot summer months our tissues and organs expand to cool the body. This alternating movement of expansion and contraction can also be recognized in the plant world. For instance, vegetation growing in a relatively cold climate is generally smaller or more compact, while the vegetation in hotter climates tends to be larger and more expanded.

These dialectical tendencies are therefore not static, but rather are always changing into one another in a continual cycle. Since they are relative tendencies, all phenomena express both yin and yang in varying degrees and characteristics; nothing is absolutely one or the other. All of nature —from the immense Milky Way galaxy right down to the elemental and subatomic realms—is organized according to a system of antagonistic yet

Fig. 1. Examples of Yin and Yang.

Tendency	Expansion	Contraction
Function	Diffusion	Fusion
	Dispersion	Assimilation
	Separation	Gathering
	Decomposition	Organization
Movement	More inactive and slower	More active and faster
Vibration	Shorter wave and high frequency	Longer wave and low frequency
Direction	Ascent and vertical	Descent and horizontal
Position	More outward and peripheral	More inward and central
Weight	Lighter	Heavier
Temperature	Colder	Hotter
Light	Darker	Brighter
Humidity	More wet	More dry
Density	Thinner	Thicker
Size	Longer	Smaller
Shape	More expansive and fragile	More contractive and harder
Form	Longer	Shorter
Texture	Softer	Harder
Atomic particle	Electron	Proton
Elements	N, O, K, P, Ca, etc.	H, C, Na, As, Mg, etc.
Environment	Vibration . . . Air . . . Water . .	. Earth
Climatic effects	Tropical climate	Colder climate
Biological	More vegetable quality	More animal quality
Sex	Female	Male
Organ structure	More hollow and expansive	More compacted and condensed
Nerves	More peripheral, ortho-sympathetic	More central, para-sympathetic
Attitude	More gentle, negative	More active, positive
Work	More psychological and mental	More physical and social
Dimension	Space	Time

* For convenience, the symbols ▽ for Yin, and △ for Yang are used.
Source: The Book of Macrobiotics, Tokyo; Japan Publications, 1977.

Fig. 2. Examples of foods as generally classified by yin and yang.

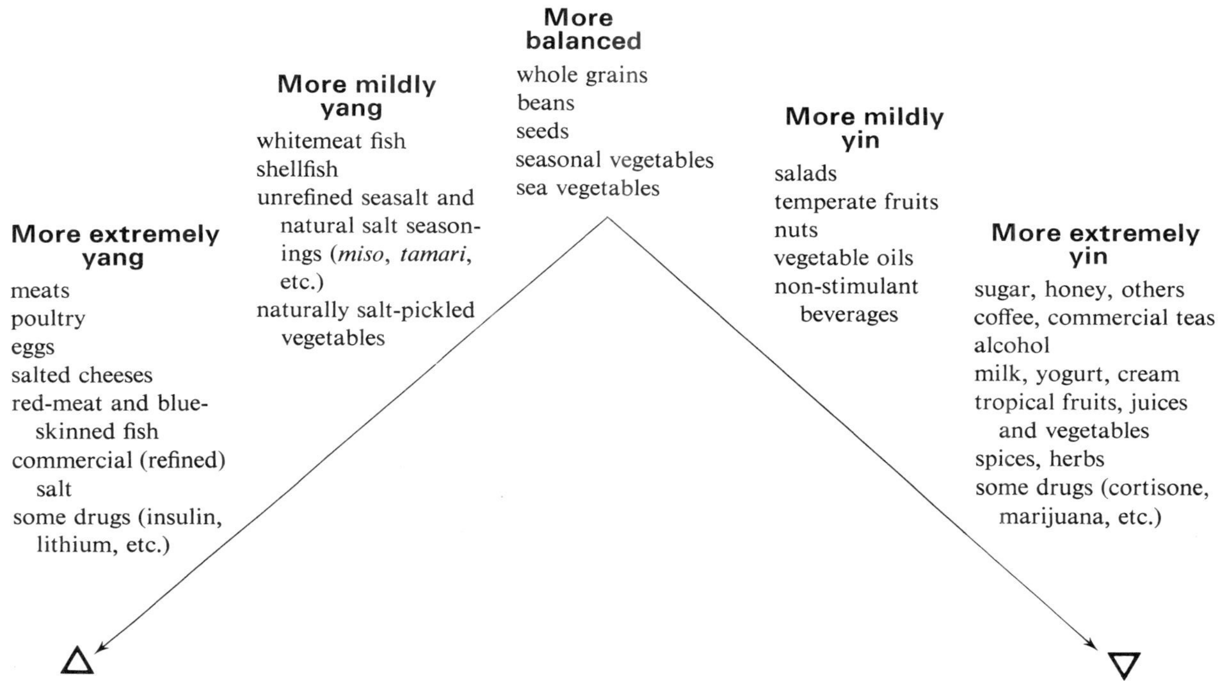

complementary qualities such as inner and outer, front and back, centripetal and centrifugal energies.

The complementary and opposite tendencies of yin and yang also exist in varying proportions and manifest physiologically as different characteristics of each food. Yin foods produce expansion of body cells, tissues, and organs, while yang foods produce contraction. Fruit is an example of a more yin food. Of the fruits, the tropical varieties are the most yin because they produce a greater expansive, cooling effect—so people tend to eat more of these during summertime. Moreover, we can also observe yin characteristics in the manner of the fruit's development. Tropical fruits grow to a relatively large size in a shorter amount of time, compared with the fruits grown in a more temperate climate. The yin force is stronger in tropical fruits, thereby allowing them to expand and grow faster. A third and more subtle way to observe the yin or yang tendency in a food is in its effects on our mentality. Strong yin food, such as sugar or ice cream, have a highly expansive and dissipating effect on our central nervous system making us feel lightheaded, spacy, or dizzy. By contrast, too much yang food has a very focusing effect, tending to give us an overly analytical, skeptical, or narrow view of life. Long-term meat eating and high salt intake can create such a yang disposition.

Macrobiotics seeks an even balance of yin and yang by avoiding extremes and emphasizing more centered foods (foods more balanced in themselves) such as whole cereal grains, beans, vegetable soups, and land and sea vegetables. The body's blood quality fluctuates constantly, like a pendulum or a seesaw. If the swing of yin and yang tendencies is too great —i.e., by eating such extremes as meat and sugar—our physiological and psychological conditions become over-stressed and weakened. The body eventually finds ways to mask or minimize the shock of these insults by storing away excess in the form of fat, or by localizations of toxins.

The Development of Sickness

Before the storing away of excess begins, the body labors to eliminate waste through a variety of physiological means, including bowel movement, urination, respiration (exhaling CO_2), and perspiration. Through these functions excessive chemical compounds are broken down into simple compounds, and ultimately, into carbon dioxide and water, which are then discharged. Normal elimination may also occur through physical, mental, and emotional activity. Mental discharge occurs in the form of wave vibrations, through our daily thoughts and expressions. Emotions such as fear or anger indicate that a great amount of excess is being discharged.

Women have the ability to discharge excess naturally through several additional channels, including menstruation, childbirth, and lactation. By these means women have a distinct advantage over men, since they can more efficiently discharge excess and thereby maintain a cleaner condition. They tend to adjust more harmoniously with their environment and usually have a longer lifespan than men. In contrast, the discharge process in men is carried out primarily by expending energy through additional physical, mental, and social activities; and men generally have a higher rate of metabolism (at rest) than women. These distinct modes of discharge operate continually throughout life. By taking in only a moderate amount of excess, they are allowed to proceed smoothly and efficiently. However, if there is overconsumption, these natural processes are not capable of fully discharging, and various abnormal processes begin.

Excessive eating and drinking, together with a disharmonious lifestyle overall, will bring about abnormal discharge, or what is often perceived as a form of physical discomfort or mild illness. This includes diarrhea, overly frequent bowel movements, excessive sweating, and excessive urination. In addition, habits like biting fingernails, scratching the head, tapping the feet, frequent blinking of the eyes, and shaky legs, also represent abnormal discharges of imbalanced energy, as do strong emotions such as fear, anger, anxiety, and depression. Wild and/or incoherent thoughts and behavior, as well as sleep often accompanied by nightmares, reflect a more acute form of discharge. Periodically, excess is discharged through violent symptoms such as coughing, sneezing, fever, shouting, crying, screaming, shivering, and trembling. All of these various forms of discharge are actually helping the body adjust to some internal imbalance which began with poor blood quality. The frequency of these various types depends on the frequency with which excess is consumed. In many cases, the continuous overburdening of our body leads to a more chronic form of discharge.

This next stage is perhaps best characterized by elimination through the skin. Skin problems are always a reflection of some internal imbalance. The chronic discharge of skin disease is an effective way to rid organs and tissues of toxins, thereby enabling them to continue more steady functioning. Skin diseases are common in cases where the kidneys have lost their ability to properly cleanse the blood stream. In modern society this usually results from heavy consumption of sugar, refined flour products, tropical fruits, and sweet beverages, as well as, alternatively, animal protein and salt. When the blood is unclean or acidic, the kidneys, heart, and all other organs begin to weaken. Besides the kidneys, another prime target organ is the liver. Proper sodium proportions, which are obtained and assimilated easiest by eating hard leafy greens, sea vegetables, and small amounts of high quality sea salt, provide the essential alkaline conditions for the liver's detoxification processes. A lack of proper dietary sodium will limit the liver's ability to filter our damaging poisons from the bloodstream. The weakening of the liver and kidneys can be detected early by various skin markings. Freckles and skin spots indicate the discharge of sugar and other refined carbohydrates, while white patches reflect the discharge of milk and dairy products. These signs may be considered indications of a tendency toward milder allergic reactions, such as skin allergy and hay fever.

If improper dietary habits still continue, then even these chronic discharge channels become sufficient. The intake of too much fat and oil, or of foods which create fat (high protein foods), may lead to a hard, dry skin condition, whereby the pores, hair follicles, and sweat glands are virtually blocked. When these blockages prevent the flow of liquids (excess) toward the surface, the skin becomes dry. The underlying layer of fat, which is preventing the usual discharge, is caused by repeated overconsumption of milk, cheese, eggs, meat, and other fatty, oily, or greasy foods. When this stage has been reached the body begins to accumulate excess. Internal deposits of mucus or fat begin to form, initially in areas that have direct access to the outside, such as the sinuses, the lower eyelids, the inner ear, and the lungs. Generally all allergic people show some sign of blockage in one or another of these areas. For example, accumulation of mucus and fat in the inner ear manifests in impaired hearing, while coughing, chest congestion, or a shallow voice all reflect accumulation in the lungs. Other areas of mucus and fat deposits include the intestines, kidneys, and sexual organs. Often, accumulation will affect these organs collectively. The heartbeat will become irregular or weak due to fatty deposits, and this is paralleled by mucus accumulation in the lungs. Not only will breathing become difficult or shallow, but the ability of the lungs to absorb oxygen and discharge carbon dioxide is substantially impeded. This, in turn, eventually weakens the oxygen-dependent filtration capacity of the kidneys, as well as the functions of other organs. In time, mucus and fat will be stored within and around the deeper, vital organs, including the heart and the liver. The more serious allergies—food allergy and allergies involving the central nervous system—are related to the more internalized forms of accumulation. These result from long-term overconsumption of hard, saturated fat, dairy food, and sugar.

Within the body, the proteins, carbohydrates, and fats that we consume often change into each other, depending on the amount of each consumed as well as the body's needs at a particular time. If we consume more of these than we need, the excess is normally discharged. However, the quantity of excess often exceeds the body's capacity to discharge it. When this happens, the excess is stored in the liver in the form of carbohydrate, in the muscles in the form of protein, or throughout the body in the form of fatty acids.

If the bloodstream is filled with fat and mucus, excess will begin to accumulate in the organs as we have seen. Since the liver and kidney are usually affected first, their functions of filtering and cleansing the blood become less efficient. This situation leads to further deterioration of the blood quality and also affects the lymphatic system. Operations such as tonsillectomies also contribute to the deterioration of the lymphatic system since they reduce the cleansing ability of this system. Such operations eventually lead to frequent swelling and lymph-gland inflammation, producing chronic deterioration of the quality of the blood, particularly the red- and white-blood cells.

Our digestive system constitutes our body's first line of defense against imbalanced or excessive foods. Poorly functioning intestines can contribute to the degeneration of blood quality since blood cells and plasma originate largely in the small intestine. Within the small intestine are millions of finger-like projections, or *villi*, which are responsible for the absorption of essential nutrients. Depending on the quality of the small intestine—as determined by the individual's quality of daily food intake—the villi will be able to either absorb proper food or reject improper, irritating food (by rapid elimination or diarrhea). In many cases, the villi of the small intestine are coated with fat and mucus, and the condition in the intestines is often acidic. Naturally, healthy blood will not be created in this type of environment.

Our blood nourishes and eventually creates the cells of our tissues and organs, including the brain. Therefore, when the blood becomes imbalanced —either too acidic or too alkaline—our metabolic functions become disharmonious. For example, overly acidic blood may lead to depression of the central nervous system, resulting in confusion, disoriented behavior, and eventually a comatose state. On the other hand, an overly alkaline condition can lead to overexcitability of the nervous system, in both the central and peripheral parts. This latter condition often manifests in muscle spasms (such as in the bronchial tubes during asthma), extreme nervousness, or convulsions. In health the blood is slightly alkaline. When its pH factor digresses from this optimum point, the body as a whole is out of balance with the natural environment. Such imbalance leads to seven general stages of sickness:

1. *Fatigue or Tiredness.* This includes both physical and mental fatigue, and can be caused by overeating, erratic exercise patterns, frequent change of occupation or residence, family problems, and so forth. At this stage, it may often be difficult to get out of bed in the morning, and the exhaustion from one day's vigorous activities may easily carry over to the next. Healthy people should be able to sleep deeply each night and always feel

fresh and energized in the morning.

One can diagnose chronic fatigue by gripping the shoulder's tightly, and also the back of the neck. If there is pain, then the muscles and circulation are overworked, and chronic fatigue has set in. One of the major causes of this prevalent problem in the modern world is the overconsumption of meat and sugar, and the lack of a whole grain-based diet.

2. *Aches and Pains.* Continual overeating and overdrinking, and lack of proper exercise, contribute to an imbalanced blood quality, as one becomes accustomed to the first stage (tiredness) and continues unhealthy living patterns. The result is occasional muscle aches, headaches, menstrual cramps, and various other minor aches; the peripheral nervous system begins to weaken and becomes slighly oversensitive, and the intercellular fluid is often highly acidic.

3. *Blood Disorders.* This stage often involves a chronically over-acid blood condition, or a fatty, sticky, or cholesterol-filled bloodstream. With this overall stagnation and chemical imbalance, skin tones, colors and textures begin to fade, becoming pale or translucent. Any of the various blood components, including antibodies, may become out of balance, leading to abnormal immune responsiveness. With a chronically poor blood condition, illnesses such as anemia, leukemia, asthma, hemophilia, jaundice, varicose veins, mononucleosis, skin diseases, leprosy, and others can easily occur. Although these may seem to be unrelated problems, their origin lies in an imbalanced blood condition and ultimately in a disorderly way of life.

4. *Emotional Disorders.* This category may involve emotions such as irritability, impatience, upset, anger, worry, fear, and uneasiness. A healthy person will not be bothered by negative emotional states, never even getting angry or feeling impatient. Emotional discharge, however, is beneficial in that it serves to release blocked excessive energy. This stage is characterized by inflammation or expansion of the peripheral nervous system, with eventual desensitization of this system. When this occurs, a person may unconsciously abuse himself with negative influences, producing chronic anxiety and frustration.

5. *Organ Diseases.* This stage marks a shift from sicknesses of adjustment to sicknesses of degeneration. It includes tuberculosis, heart disease, diabetes, various allergies, emphysema, ulcers, cirrhosis of the liver, and gallstones. As the body continues to collect excess toxins, fat, and mucus, it attempts to store and localize the harmful substances in certain areas.

However, there is a threshold beyond which this localizing process cannot proceed without causing pain or impairing organ function. This stage may also include infection and/or some deficiency in immune functions.

6. *Nerve Diseases.* At this point, if the body has succeeded in masking the expression of excess, various types of mental illness, multiple sclerosis, Parkinson's disease, and different types of paralysis may occur. The individual's psychological orientation becomes disharmonious, sometimes producing dullness, forgetfullness, manic depression, and violent social behavior. As the sensory nervous system becomes increasingly dulled the central nervous system begins to lose its integral sense of relationship with the universe.

7. *Arrogance.* In time, with continued disharmonious living, the central nervous system becomes highly resistant and non-cooperative with the environment, and there is strong energetic and biochemical stagnation overall. When this happens, we try to separate ourselves from nature and the universe.

The larger purpose of macrobiotic healing, therefore, is to dissolve arrogance. Modern medicine can relieve a broad spectrum of symptoms, as can acupuncture and other forms of traditional medical technique; but these more symptomatic approaches do not address this basic problem of arrogance, which we may also define as a sense of complete separation from the benign environment, whether expressed on physical, physiological or psychological levels.

Sickness can also be classified as diseases of adjustment or of degeneration. Stages one through four of the above categories can be classified as adjustment illnesses, while stages five through seven are degenerative. As we will see later, allergy is associated with both the fourth and fifth stages.

1. *Sicknesses of Adjustment.* This type of illness often occurs after someone who has been eating in a balanced way suddenly begins to eat in an imbalanced way, and develops diarrhea, stomach pains, fever, or vomiting. Such symptoms are often labeled as sicknesses, but, in fact, are nothing but the natural, healthy elimination of poisons or toxins. Another example is *tonsillitis*, which happens when the lymphatic system tries to localize toxins and acids generated by improper diet. In this case, the accompanying fever is only an attempt to "burn off" excess. Through such adjustments, we are able to maintain a more neutral or balanced condition.

Another example of an adjustment is irregular menstruation. This occurs because a woman is eating unbalanced food, such as meat or other animal foods. People who eat these types of food also often experience an unpleasant body odor. This again reflects the body's attempt to eliminate excess, as shown also by skin diseases, headaches, and discharges of various other types. It is usually better not to interfere with the discharge process unless it is very acute. Symptoms disappear when the excess has been eliminated completely. By eating very well during this process, the body remains strong, and self-healing abilities develop easily. Adjustments like these need not be considered as actual illnesses.

2. *Degenerative Sicknesses.* Degenerative ailments may actually be considered as true sicknesses, since they are created by chronic deterioration of a variety of physiological functions. Some types of degenerative illness arise when the body's cells begin to decompose into their primitive, pre-cellular forms. Cells are originally created by the aggregation and fusion of millions of bacteria, and when the reverse process occurs, this is considered an infectious disease.

After eating properly for a few years the body is able to dispose of any unnatural excess. When such a person eats a hot dog for example, he will often vomit or have diarrhea soon afterward. This arises because the hot dog is not a natural human food. Therefore, as our condition improves through proper eating, we become increasingly sensitive to the effects of all food. If we don't experience some reaction after eating imbalanced food, we are accumulating excess and our condition is degenerating. Some of us can do this for 20 years or longer without any external symptoms, and we may not be aware of how our overall body functioning, including our judgment, is gradually becoming more dull the longer we eat in an unnatural manner. People in this condition often find it difficult to understand why they should eat a balanced diet. In many cases, their orientation is something like: "I have been eating meat for 40 years and am in perfect health, so why should I change now?" However, this type of person often has a sudden heart attack or may, apparently without warning, eventually abruptly develop cancer, diabetes or another life threatening problem.

The mechanism of sickness may also be viewed in terms of the difference between *condition* and *constitution.* Our condition is a result of our day-to-day eating patterns, and is therefore always changing. On the other hand, our constitution changes at an extremely gradual and almost imperceptible rate. Constitution can be thought of as one's original natal condition. In other words, constitution represents our prenatal condition as determined by our mother's diet during pregnancy. After birth, this becomes our constitution, which continues to be formed until about the age of 22 for women and 24 for men. This process is completed with the appearance of wisdom teeth. In general, adjustments represent changes in condition, while degenerative diseases affect constitution.

Macrobiotics and Human Freedom

When we reflect deeply on our relationship with the outer world, our environment, we realize that we are never independent of its influences. In a broad sense, everything is food: the air, light and sound waves, electromagnetic radiation, the quality of vibration emitted from the clothes we wear, and of course, the food on our table. How we select from this magnificent world of energy determines the quality of our human condition. Physical food is the part of our environment over which we exercise the most control, and through which we establish our ability to receive non-physical food or vibration. In other words, by creating a strong biological foundation through proper dietary practice one may obtain the capacity for greater adaptability, broader thinking and a more universal awareness. For the majority of people, such rewards would seem only possible by many years of meditation practice, elaborate education, or esoteric mental disciplines. However, these measures are often impractical and perhaps inappropriate for many people in the modern world. Instead, we can create a harmonious life of endless play in our own home, and in our own family by simply creating a balanced daily life. Freeing ourselves from the limitations that allergies impose, in fact, is often only the first step in freeing ourselves from self-limitations on other levels, leading to the progressive development of human freedom. This is the purpose of macrobiotics.

2. The Riddle of Allergies

The History of Allergies

In the early days of the science of immunology, immunity and allergy were viewed as having an opposite, complementary relationship, like two sides of the same coin. The two sides could be called "tolerance" and "intolerance." In terms of tolerance or immunity, the body's immune system is normally able to overcome foreign intruders (the invading virus, bacteria, etc.) and, in the process, becomes educated for future resistance to these intruders. This process is also called *immunization* or *desensitization*, since it involves an individual becoming less adversely sensitive to a potentially harmful substance. All organisms or foreign substances are therefore dealt with in an orderly manner, with no dramatic or abnormal body signals. In the case of intolerance or allergy, the body's natural defense forces overreact to the intruders, and to all kinds of normally harmless, non-toxic substances. The result is a violent resistance to these foreign elements, and the subsequent weakening of body functions as a whole.

The process of immunization or desensitization, that is, of inducing tolerance, has been recognized by traditional wisdom for a long time. Certain groups of American Indians consumed small portions of poison ivy or poison oak to become immune to their toxic and irritating effects, and some wild food foragers still maintain this practice today. There are stories of farmers who would feed their goats the poisonous plants and then drink their milk to receive immunity. One recorded instance of immunization dates back to the ancient king Mithridates, who reigned over a land that later became Persia. Fearing that someone might poison him to usurp his huge kingdom, the king began taking small doses of poisons to build tolerance to them. So tells the poet, A. E. Housman:

> He gathered all that springs to birth
> From the many-venomed earth;
> First a little, thence to more,
> He sampled all her killing store . . .
> —I tell the tale that I heard told.
> Mithridates, he died old.

In a similar way, doctors today desensitize a person to the things to which he or she is allergic. Allergy shots are regularly given to gradually innoculate an individual with the very elements that cause a reactions.

Ronald Reagan, for example, who is allergic to house dust, animal danders, feathers, outdoor pollens, burlap and some of the stuffed antique relics in the White House, receives desensitization shots on a weekly basis. Julias Caesar also had allergies, although there are no written accounts as to how he dealt with the ailment.

The history of allergy extends back to ancient times. In 3000 B.C., Shen Nung, the emperor of China, ruled that pregnant woman should not eat fish, chicken, or horse meat, since these foods sometimes appeared to cause sudden ulceration of the skin. According to some scholars, many of the dietary restrictions mentioned in the Old Testament were formulated because it was observed that certain foods brought about strong reactions.

Some of the well-known early Greek physicians also appear to have had encounters with the illness. In the second century A.D., Galen described people who could not help sneezing when exposed to certain plants. Hippocrates provided perhaps the earliest accounts of asthma and milk allergy, and wrote, "It is a bad thing to give milk to persons having headache." There is also the famous statement by Lucretius, from the first century B.C., that "one man's meat is another man's poison." Of course, he may have been referring to differences in individual responses to foods that were not necessarily allergy-related. But the basic understanding of susceptibility was there.

Modern immunology actually began with the first pioneering studies of allergic phenomena. Throughout the 1800's, British physicians described a number of hay fever, asthma, and other allergic cases. Then, in 1902, two Frenchmen, Portier and Richet, were hired to study the Portugese Man-O'-War, a jellyfish, for Prince Albert of Monaco. By injecting the sea creature's poison into dogs, they tried to implant immunity. To their surprise, however, the poison gave no reaction on the first injection, but proved severely toxic, and often fatal, when injected a second time, one to three weeks after the first injection. Richet named this phenomenon *anaphylaxis*, from the Greek roots: *ana* meaning "without" and *phylaxis* meaning "protection." The term was intended to convey the opposite of protection. The French scientists attributed the bizarre reaction of the dogs to a loss of immunity due to the first injection, so that the second injection had fatal results. Somehow, the phenomenon of tolerance had changed into extreme intolerance. Soon after, this phenomenon was observed in susceptible animals with ordinary, non-toxic substances.

One of the most notable attempts of the early 1900's to clarify the relationship between allergy and food came from the careful research of a British psychiatrist, Dr. Francis Hare. In 1906, Dr. Hare published an immense book—a thousand pages long and in two volumes—called *The Food Factor in Disease*. In these volumes he declared that bronchitis, asthma, eczema, various digestive disorders, angina, high blood pressure, gout, migraine, epilepsy, arthritis, and a number of other illnesses were caused by the patient eating an excess of sugary or refined high-starch foods. He observed that patients whose diets consisted largely of sugary, starchy foods would improve dramatically when these carbohydrates were reduced or removed from the diet. If the patients started eating sugary, starchy foods soon afterwards, the old problems would resurface. Dr. Hare was also fascinated by withdrawal symptoms of intense irritability and malaise, which often happened with patients who stopped consuming sugary foods. This "addictive phase" would disappear when people were able to avoid the foods for several days or more. Today's allergists and nutritionists know that not all sugar "addictions" are associated with allergies; some are instead related to other aspects of an individual's dietary practice, such as the extent of salt- and meat-eating.

In the same year that Hare published his great book, Dr. Clement Von Pirquet, an Austrian pediatrician, introduced the term *allergy* as a replacement for anaphylaxis. The word *allergy* stemmed from two Greek words, *allos* meaning "altered" or "other," and *ergon* meaning "work" or "action." In other words, allergy was originally viewed as a state of altered reactivity. Von Pirquet hypothesized that altered states of reactivity were triggered by the arrival of a foreign substance, or *antigen*. The hyperreactive response seemed to depend on whether an antigen had previously been introduced to the immune system. However, the successors of Von Pirquet soon realized that previous sensitization did not necessarily mean that anaphylaxis would occur. On the contrary, several possibilities arose:

1) Healthy immune response, with neutralization and disposal of the potential offender or foreign substance;
2) Paralysis or switching off of the immune system as a passive means of tolerance;
3) Abnormal immune response or allergy. We can interpret these three responses as representing a scale of physiological health, from more balanced (1), to more yin and weakened (2), and finally to a very extreme yin, weakened condition (3) with the exaggerated, overly yang compensating reactions that sometimes accompany allergies.

Since the time of Von Pirquet, science has searched for the factors that determine which of these three possibilities will manifest. The Austrian physician had identified only the mechanical prerequisite for allergy—previous exposure or sensitization.

Since allergy means a state of altered reactivity, it occurs only in certain individuals. While one person may react abnormally to something in the

Fig. 3. Degrees of immune response.

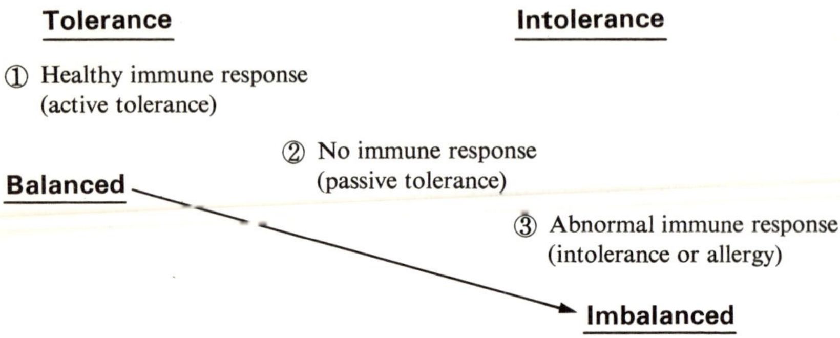

environment, another is apparently not affected. With the development of the field of immunology, the mechanisms of allergic reactions have received almost exclusive attention since they are thought to be related to a number of disease states, including cancer and various infectious diseases. Relatively little research, however, has addressed the more fundamental cause-and-effect relationships of allergy. According to the conventional view, the only preventive approach is to counteract the more superficial causes—the allergens such as pollen, animal dander, and so on. Therefore, the primary question remains unanswered: Why are certain individuals more prone to allergic tendencies than others? Or stated another way: "Why isn't everyone allergic?"

The idea of allergy as the body's inability to tolerate the environment was eventually modified by a more specialized explanation. From advanced microscopic studies developed over the past 15 years, the new view of allergy has become confined to an abnormal antigen-antibody reaction. Unfortunately, this narrow redefinition has neglected to address the issue of susceptibility. At best, it has again viewed susceptibility in terms of poorly understood genetic tendencies, even though the supporting evidence for this view is vague and inconsistent. In cases where no hereditary link or offending antigen could be found, psychological factors have often been suspected as the cause of hypersensitivity.

In response to this confusion, an entirely new school of thought called *clinical ecology* has emerged. According to the "ecologists," the immunological explanation must be revised to account for a wide range of allergic disorders, both physical and mental, which are evoked by foods and environmental chemicals. The idea is that certain foods or food additives consumed over a long period of time will often lead to an individual's inability to tolerate these foods. Some clinical ecologists have proposed that the toxic substances entering the food chain in industrial countries may be causing degeneration of the immune system, leading to abnormal responses such as allergy. One controversial hypothesis of the ecologists is that food allergy may actually underlie many common allergies, as well as a vast array of other illnesses, including arthritis, epilepsy, cancer, and heart disease.

The Role of the Environment

The fact that environmental factors contribute strongly to *atopic* (allergic) disease is well documented. Diet and lifestyle are now recognized as the most important influences in one's susceptibility to allergy in early life, although the relationship is still largely misunderstood: the conventional emphasis is on food allergy developed during pregnancy and childhood as a result of allergenic foods eaten by the mother and/or growing child. Sensitization of the fetus and newborn to cow's milk proteins can occur both prenatally and during breastfeeding. This may occur in spite of the fact that the mother herself shows no biochemical evidence of similar hypersensitivity to cow's milk. Other interesting factors are the time of birth and level of economic development. Children born in late autumn or early winter tend to develop asthma more often than children born at other times of the year. Atopic disorders are less common in developing countries than in industrial countries. These observations point to a fundamental relationship between various environmental factors and the physiology of allergy.

As allergies have continued to afflict increasing numbers of people in the modern world, modern science has been compelled to restructure its conceptions of the disease. The clinical ecologists believe that allergy has evolved out of the adverse environmental effects of modern industrialization. Chemicals and toxins in our food, water, air, cosmetics, drugs, etc., have encouraged a weakening of the body's normal homeostatic functions. The high incidence of allergy in the United States is but a small sample reflection of this biological breakdown, showing that our natural immunity is becoming "artificialized," or that our inherent body wisdom is becoming deranged. This view was echoed by Rachel Carson's *Silent Spring*, in which she discussed the sensitizing and toxic effects of insecticides, pesticides, herbicides, and other commonly used industrial chemicals. Carson pointed out various differences regarding individual susceptibility and allergic tendencies; for example, that women appear to be more susceptible than men, younger people more than adults, and those who lead sedentary, indoor lives more than those who lead active, outdoor lives. Besides these basic distinctions, Carson called the reasons behind individual sensitivity a "medical mystery." However, she went on to point out that many of these chemicals, when ingested or inhaled, could have extremely harmful effects on the liver, kidneys, and nervous system—all of which appear to be intimately involved in abnormal sensitivity or intolerance. Other prominent figures, like Alexis Carrel and Rene Dubos, have explored the meaning of adaptation—both physical and mental—in the context of modernized living conditions. Both men view these conditions as conducive to the decay of adaptive functions, including our natural immunity or overall resistance. On the surface at least, allergy seems to reflect an aberration in man's adaptive responsiveness to the increasing artificialization of his environment.

Obviously, we cannot ignore the many influences of our polluted environment (especially food) and over-abundant lifestyle. The average American eats nine pounds of chemical additives a year, including preservatives, flavoring agents, stabilizers, and artificial colors. Over 3,000 synthetic and natural chemicals are now used for preserving, coloring, flavoring and stabilizing prepared foods—this amounts to about $485,000,000 worth of food additives each year. The standard loaf of white bread contains benzoyl peroxide bleach, tricalcium phosphate (to make flour run smoothly), potassium bromate (maturing agent), calcium propitionate (to prevent molds), and a choice of about 10 preservatives. This is in addition to refined wheat flour, milk, eggs, yeast, water, vegetable oil(s), iodized salt, sugar, and an array of synthetic vitamins.

Half a century ago the standard homemade loaf consisted simply of whole wheat flour, salt, water, and usually a little yeast. This comparatively wholesome food was eaten within a day or two of baking, whereas today's version may sit on the shelf for weeks, gradually absorbing chemicals or synthetic gasses from the plastic or cellophane wrapper. Moreover, what goes on top of the bread is also loaded: Today's butter contains synthetic hormones (from the cow's diet), bright yellow dye, penicillin, added minerals and synthetic vitamins, fish oil, citrus juice, and alcohol solvent. Food technology is not only transforming familiar foods, but is creating entirely new ones, with various colors, flavors, and textures to appeal to the sensorial whims of the public. Pre-made frozen dinners, canned desserts, powdered juice bases, and numerous other products are created, dried, pulverized, sprayed, cooked or frozen at some distant factory to be stored indefinitely. Eventually one of these up to eight year old contrivances will reach the dinner table, often to be gobbled down with a soda or coffee.

As each new chemical additive enters the food market, an increasing risk is imposed on the health of the consumer. Many of these additives are untested for side-effects, or only given very limited, inadequate testing. Moreover, the identification of certain additives (such as food colorings) on food labels is usually unclear or misleading. For example, the presence of coloring in butter, cheese, and ice cream need not be specified at all, according to the Food and Drug Administration (FDA). In other foods, colorings are only identified generally as "artificial coloring," giving people the false impression that there is probably only one dye, or that no variation exists among the greens, blues, oranges, etc. Because of this ambiguity, a person who is allergic to one food coloring is compelled to avoid all foods containing artificial coloring. (Such allergies may surely prove beneficial in the long-term!) Lastly, the information provided by the manufacturers concerning the food additives' side-effects is not only scant, but quite likely inaccurate: It fails to take into account the interaction (*synergistic* effect) produced by the additive's combination with other substances in the food. The risk of introducing additional unfamiliar chemicals into our system is dangerous beyond comprehension, yet few people are willing to replace the mass-produced, convenience food for good quality, natural whole food.

One often overlooked risk of the modern food situation is the inclusion of presumably "safe" food components, and the processing of known safe foods. Taking the example of the standard supermarket loaf, we observe in addition to many additives, a list of regular bread ingredients including refined wheat flour, milk, eggs, yeast, iodized salt, sugar, and synthetic vitamins. All of these are generally assumed to be normal or even necessary, but this is a misconception. Refined wheat flour is depleted of valuable vitamins (particularly B-vitamins, which are essential to the integrity of the immune and nervous systems), as well as of proteins and minerals. To compensate for this, the bread is fortified with these and other nutrients that are naturally present in whole wheat flour. The National Academy of Sciences has recently pointed out that adding vitamins to foods often produces covert toxic effects, and that, therefore, whole unadulterated foods should be preferred. Moreover, added vitamins do not cancel the effects of various additives or sugar; surprisingly, to the contrary, they enhance the effects of these other components. Sugar itself will deplete the body's supply of B- and D-vitamins, gradually paralyze the nervous system, acidify the blood (leading to fatigue), and impair the functions of various organs, particularly the spleen, pancreas, stomach and kidneys. Commercial milk and eggs contain an excess of protein, simple carbohydrate, fat, and various chemicals (synthetic hormones, etc.). These foods, in addition to yeast, will also interfere with normal digestive assimilation. The iodized salt is virtually devoid of trace minerals and thus has very little nutritional value. Finally, the combination of milk, sugar, and additives is fundamental to the development of allergy.

Four basic aspects of the standard modern diet have contributed to widespread biological degeneration:

(1) The lack of essential nutrients because of processing, and weakening digestive functions;

(2) The imbalanced proportions of other nutrients due to fortification and improper food combinations;
(3) Food additives or toxins;
(4) The declining quality (freshness and revitalizing potential) of available animal and vegetable products due to the extensive use of agricultural and marketing chemicals, processing, and so on.

On top of this, our biological systems must endure the stresses of densely populated living conditions, industrial pollution, and often harmful or weakening medical treatments. The organ of our body that is primarily affected by all of these stresses, including chemically processed food, is the liver. This great metabolic mastermind controls and regulates the quantity, the quality, and the use of the foods we take in. Overall, the liver acts on the blood and its contents to monitor the quality of the internal environment—by dispensing with various bodily excesses—and to neutralize unwanted or poisonous substances. The liver attempts to lessen various forms of unnatural physiological stress, including pollutants, food additives, medicines, drugs, alcohol, and other chemicals (caffeine, nicotine, etc.). Doctors for example have to administer a large enough dose of aspirin so that no matter how hard the liver works to prevent it from entering the bloodstream, enough aspirin enters to do the symptomatic job. Another harmful practice is overeating (of any food) as well as eating less balanced foods. Flour products, fruit, milk, dairy products, meat, oil and fat all result in mucus and fat build-up in the liver. The consequent degradation of its thousands of regulatory functions opens the doors for degeneration elsewhere in the body. Along with the breakdown of liver functions, mucus and fat deposits in the kidneys and lungs, and later in the spleen and lymphatic channels, will strongly predispose one to allergy or other changes in immune responsiveness.

Many doctors and allergists know such degeneration is occurring, and many have subsequently recommended adequate rest, exercise, and good nutrition. Unfortunately there is a general lack of understanding about nutrition. Moreover, as with the clinical ecologists, the issue of abnormal sensitivity has clouded the issue of the root cause. Allergists are inclined to view foods and food components based more on their *allergenicity* (their ability to elicit an allergic reaction) than anything else. Thus the conventional view of environments in regard to allergy has become: "To what are we sensitive and how much?" As opposed to: "What makes us sensitive in the first place?"

Fortunately, the former view is not entirely without merit. Foods like milk and eggs are recognized as some of the most potent allergenic foods around. Therefore many allergists are now recommending that they be avoided, even when no overt or clinical evidence for hypersensitivity is found. Also, the potential degenerating and sensitizing effect of additives and hidden chemicals within foods have led a number of top allergy specialists to advocate natural, unadulterated foods. One of the more negative aspects of this focus on allergenicity, however, is the occasional incrimination of perfectly healthful foods, such as whole cereal grains and legumes, which are sometimes involved in food allergy.

The Immunological View

When people talk about immunity they are usually referring to the body's overall protection against disagreeable symptoms. In the field of law, the term denotes exemption from legal obligations or freedom from liability. As defined by modern medicine, however, immunity is not to be associated in any sense with complete or absolute freedom. Medical practitioners refer to immunity as a state of lessened susceptibility to injury by microorganisms and by certain poisons formed by animals and plants—a state of protection that may rise to a peak in response to an attack (or to some stimulus) and may lapse at other times. Unfortunately, this variability in immunological competence perplexes many medical scientists, since the highly specialized field of immunology has limited itself to the complex microscopic mechanism of the immune response. It has neglected to explore the reasons for immunological variability both within the individual and between individuals. Such an inquiry calls for an understanding of the human organism as an integrated whole, and as inseparable from the environment upon which its life depends.

Modern physiology recognizes that the human body is endowed with a certain degree of *natural* immunity—innate resistance to infection by microorganisms or invasion by their toxins. Natural immunity is a more generalized dimension of the body's entire defense system. Immunologists primarily view natural immunity in terms of certain blood components. Our blood is composed of a great variety of substances that act directly on microorganisms or their toxins to destroy or inactivate them. Some of these are for example: 1) *lysozyme*, a polysaccharide that dissolves certain bacteria; 2) *interferon*, a large protein that inactivates many viruses; 3) *properdin*, another large protein that acts directly to destroy certain bacteria (*gram-negative* bacteria); and 4) certain basic proteins that similarly react with other kinds of bacteria (*gram-positive* bacteria). These constitute only a minute sampling of the many materials circulating in our blood which contribute to natural immunity. In times of illness—such as during the early stages of fever—before specific antibodies appear—the power of killing certain bacteria is much increased. Thus during sickness the blood has an amazing capacity to respond appropriately for immediate protection.

In addition, natural immunity includes the overall protection which results from general processes directed at specific disease organisms or substances. Four simplified examples are as follows:

1) The resistance of the skin—the body's main physical barrier—to all kinds of infection. The skin secretes antiseptic substances in the sweat. This minimizes the survival chances of potentially infectious agents.
2) The destruction of unwanted foreign organisms by the stomach's acid secretions and digestive enzymes.
3) The lymph system, which "cleans" the blood, though the recognition and ingestion (*phagocytosis*) of invading organisms by white blood cells and *reticuloendothelial* cells (distributed throughout the tissue linings of blood and lymph channels).
4) The metabolic detoxification of many toxic compounds and drugs by the liver.

Other aspects of natural immunity include the essential functions of the excretory system and autonomic nervous system. As we will see, preserving the biological integrity of these systems is critical for the prevention of allergic disorders.

In addition to natural immunity—the body's primary line of defense—we also have a so-called *acquired immunity* in response to certain environmental stimuli, such as microorganisms and viruses and their toxins, foreign tissues (from surgical operations), and a vast number of other substances. This second system, which has also been called *adaptive immunity*, is entirely complementary to the body's natural immunity. They are actually just two sides of the coin of immunity. Acquired immunity is distinguished as a finer tuning of our physiological defenses; it provides highly specific immune reactions to foreign organisms to which the body does not appear to have natural immunity. For example, upon first exposure to a foreign substance, the body may not be able to block or neutralize it. However, within a few days to a few weeks after exposure, the immune system usually develops powerful and specific resistance to that particular substance; this is an example of acquired immunity.

Traditionally, acquired immunity has been separated, into two distinct parts: *humoral* and *cellular*. In the humoral type the body produces circulating disease-fighting proteins, the antibodies, which respond specifically to the introduction of a foreign agent or *antigen*. This type of acquired immunity may take weeks or even months to appear following the antigen's initial entry. In the other type of acquired immunity it is not the production of circulating proteins elicited by antigen, but rather the highly specialized lymph cells derived from the thymus. After initial contact with the anti-

Fig. 4. Natural and acquired (humoral and cellular) immunity.

①Natural Immunity:

immediate, more general response.

1. Blood components
2. Lymph
3. Skin
4. Liver and stomach
5. Excretory and autonomic nervous systems

②Acquired Immunity:

more long-term, specific, fine-tuned response.

Lymph

Humoral (▽)
circulating antibodies

Cellular (△)
localized antibodies

genic substance, the lymphocytes become sensitized and later attach to the antigenic agent to neutralize it.

Our acquired immunity is the product of the body's lymphatic tissue. The lymphatic system consists of lymph capillaries, vessels, ducts and nodes which are present throughout the body and in most internal organs, particularly the spleen and tonsils. The function of the *lymphatics* (lymph channels) is to transport *lymph fluid*—that portion of the blood which leaks out of the circulatory system due to the enormous pressure the blood is under. The *lymph* is a clear fluid which accumulates in the tissue spaces —between the cells and blood capillaries—and eventually enters the lymphatic network. Unlike blood which is circulated by the pumping motion of the heart, the lymph is moved by several factors: the normal contraction of nearby muscles during physical activity; the contraction of the lungs and diaphragm during breathing; and the movements of the villi and the contractions of the small intestine.

The bloodstream is considered more yang since its main function is to transport the iron-rich red blood cells. The lymph system, consisting primarily of white blood cells which are larger than red blood cells, and bear a slightly negative charge, is more yin. Both comprise the circulatory system as a whole and circulate in opposite yet complementary directions. Blood circulation begins in the heart, radiates outward to the more peripheral regions, and then returns. Conversely, the flow of lymph begins in the peripheral body tissues and then re-enters the general circulation near the heart region.

While the lymph fluid is moving toward the heart region, it passes through many tiny bean-shaped glands called *lymph nodes*. These minute concentrated masses of lymphatic tissue act as primary filters, protecting the bloodstream from numerous external substance. Each node contains scavenger cells, for example, *macrophages* and reticuloendothelial cells which ingest and destroy disease organisms. When certain parts of our body become infected, the lymph nodes will draw lymph from the infected area, and may subsequently swell and become tender. Special lymphatic tissue with similar neutralizing potential is found in the spleen, in "patches" along the intestines, and, to a slight extent, in the bone marrow. The lymphatic tissues collectively constitute a fine protective network which, in healthy individuals, is virtually invincible to the immense variety of foreign, unwanted organisms or toxins which can enter our circulation.

The lymphatic tissue is the source of antibody production. When an antigen enters the body it is engulfed and broken down by a macrophage, which then relays the news to a lymphocyte. At this point the information transferred may pertain to the required specificity of the antibody. The lymphocyte then differentiates into a plasma cell which begins producing antibodies of the required specificity. The whole process may take a week or longer, and presumably results in either one of two possible immune responses, as mentioned previously. One is humoral, whereby antibodies are released into the bloodstream, often to neutralize a foreign substance, or to avert bacterial and viral infections. In allergic persons, the humoral response is called an *immediate hypersensitivity*, since the reaction happens rapidly. The other type is cellular, in which antibodies remain within a sensitized lymphocyte. This type is also referred to an *delayed hypersensitivity* because reactions take longer than those of humoral antibodies. Delayed hypersensitivity is the primary response in most viral, protozoal, fungal, and in some bacterial infections.

Fig. 5. Humoral and cellular phases of immune response.

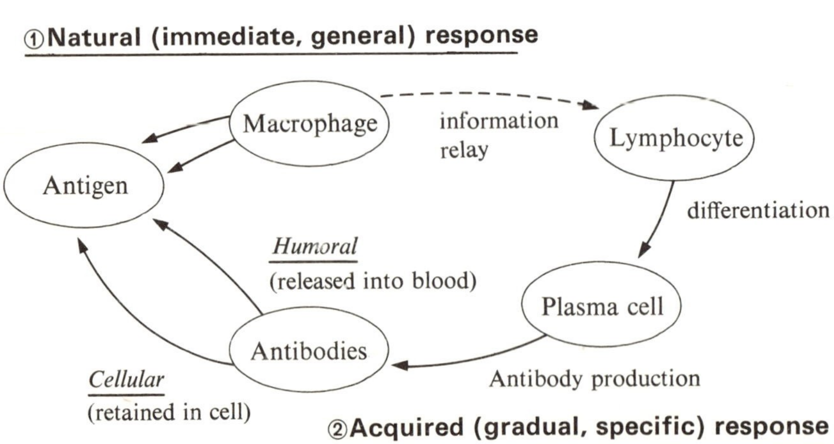

The New View of the Immune System

Historically, the immune system has been analyzed in terms of either humoral or cellular reactions. Recently, however, as a result of extensive assimilation and reorganization of immunological data, a new understanding has evolved which integrates the two mechanisms. Briefly, this perspective can be described as follows. Two kinds of circulating lymphyocytes, *T-cells* and *B-cells*, are derived from undifferentiated cells which originate in the embryonic yolk sac. T-cells, which mainly participate in delayed hypersensitivity reactions, are converted to functional status by the thymus gland. B-cells, which have a more direct role in allergic responses, are formed primarily by lymphoid tissues of the intestines (including the appendix), spleen, and liver. According to the new model, the immune response to almost all antigens involves the cooperation of the two types of lymphocytes. Thus, the B-cell is converted into an antibody-producing plasma cell by the cooperative action of activated T-cells, in addition to direct stimulation by the antigen.

The production of two distinct types of lymphocytes from the undifferentiated stem cell is critical to the immunologic integrity of those cells. By this process, the B- and T-cells become intimately interwoven in all immune reactions. These lymphocytes share a complementary and antagonistic relationship, as reflected by the variation in their size, density, lifespan, and overall functioning. The B-cell is governed by the more centrifugal (yin) force, while the T-cell is governed by the more centripetal (yang) force. This classification is obtained by the following comparisons:

B-cell	T-cell
More diffuse or expanded structure	More dense or compact structure
More stationary and passive	More mobile and aggressive (there are helper, suppressor, and even "killer" T-cells)
"Memory" is induced slowly in response to antigen	Memory is induced quickly in response to antigen
Shorter lifespan (more delicate)	Longer lifespan (more durable)
Carry many long microvilli (tiny hairs) on celi surface	Carry fewer and shorter microvilli on cell surface
Activation by antigen causes cell to expand then differentiate	Activation by antigen does not cause cell to expand nor differentiate

Following their production within the B-cell, antibodies are externalized, then enter the general circulation	Following their production within the T-cell, antibodies are retained permanently inside the cell
Are processed by several large organs—the intestines, liver, and spleen.	Are processed by one small organ, the thymus.
Are found in loose, more dispersed spirallic formation in the spleen	Are found in tight, more dense sprallic clusters in the spleen

When the immune system is out of balance, the integral relationship between the humoral and cellular components, the B- and T-cells respectively, becomes upset. Macrobiotics provides a practical understanding of how this imbalance is created on the macroscopic level, through an imbalance in the yin and yang aspects of one's diet and daily life. Within this understanding lies the key to the true relief of allergy, and the profound enjoyment of sound health.

The Issue of Genetics

Modern immunology holds that allergic disorders are probably intricately related to *immunodeficiency diseases*—those diseases which appear as a result of a faulty development of the immune system and immune responsiveness. The central tenet of this perspective is that genetic defects lead to various deficiencies in the normal or acquired immune mechanisms. These defects may either be *pure* (singular) or *mixed* (multiple). The pure defects may involve either specific lymph cell production, or antibody synthesis, or phagocytosis. Mixed defects, on the other hand, may involve the deficiency of any combination of these mechanisms. Other defects include deficiencies of *complement* (substances which seem to direct the binding of antibody and antigen) or enzymes needed to activate the complement system.

While it is conceivable that genetic defects take place at certain stages in the development of immunologic mechanisms (thus determining when and how the deficiency will manifest), there is a general lack of understanding as to why these defects might occur in the first place. In other words, what factors determine when genetic flaws will be expressed or whether they will be expressed at all? Unfortunately, there has been very little communication between the rapidly developing fields of immunology, genetics and nutrition. It is well established, however, that acquired immune disorders in humans occur with deficiencies of iron, zinc, vitamin A, vitamin B_6, vitamin B_{12}, and folic acid, and with excesses of essential fatty acids and vitamin E. Other micronutrients and trace elements, and the quality of fats, proteins, and carbohydrates, must be provided in proper balance to create immunological harmony.

How can food influence the immune system if abnormalities result from genetic defects? There is now considerable evidence for a dynamic communication between the cell's cytoplasmic factors and the genetic material of the nucleus. Furthermore, the DNA molecules are in a constant state of flux, always expanding and contracting, and replacing bits of information along their helical chains; and these changes in the DNA are related to changes in the intercellular fluid composition. Our cells are therefore capable of "inheriting" new information from their environment; and the intercellular environment itself is ultimately derived from the food we eat. Placed in this perspective, genetic mechanisms, which are operating throughout our lifetimes to direct billions of physiological functions, are not so mysterious and inaccessible as once thought to be. The more basic flaw may lie more in our own judgment—and the way of life we choose to practice.

In order to understand the phenomenon of allergy we must look beyond what antibodies and antigens are doing to why they are doing it. Since allergies often "run in the family," a hereditary cause has been emphasized, even though the evidence supporting a hereditary predisposition is circumstantial, and there it still no known genetic mechanism compatible with the existing scientific data. Consider the relative incidence of allergy in identical twins: while one may develop allergy, the other may never develop the condition. One way we can more clearly understand allergy is to explore the fundamental nature of antibodies and antigens—their origins, make-up, and the kind of environment which favors their production and activity.

Antibodies and Antigens: Enemies or Friends?

Allergies which involve the interaction between antibodies and antigens are the primary focus of allergy research in this country. Generally speaking, antibodies, as well as the sensitized lymphocytes (either B- or T-cells), have a more primary causal role in allergy than do antigens. An organism, toxin, or any substance in the environment may be termed antigenic because it contains one or more specific chemical compounds in its make-up which appear to initiate an acquired immune response. Antigens generally consist of certain proteins, large *polysaccharides* (chains of simple sugars), or large *lipoprotein* (fat plus protein) complexes. Almost all bacteria and their toxins are composed of strongly antigenic chemical compounds, and there are literally billions of potentially antigenic materials in nature. It is therefore a true wonder that the human body is capable of recognizing each antigen and dealing with it appropriately. How the immune system maintains this tremendous adaptability—the ability to produce the necessary antibody for the infinite range of possible antigens—is one of the greatest mysteries of the human body.

Antibodies, on the other hand, are simply a class of proteins which circulate in the blood, playing a key role in most immune responses. Proteins have been identified structurally as *globulin*, hence the term *immunoglobulins*. The job of antibodies is to neutralize, through chemical and electromagnetic means, foreign organisms or substances which enter the body. Part of every antibody's structure are certain molecules which interlock with the outer covering of the antigen. To complete this jigsaw-like interlocking, certain other blood proteins (complement) coat the antibody-antigen complex. The complex is then ready to be eaten by the phagocytic cells of the lymph system, or is effectively neutralized and excreted through the bile or feces, or is destroyed directly by complement. This is the general course of the normal immune response.

The key to this process is the principle of the attraction of yin and yang: each antibody complements and therefore binds with the antigen whose precise proportions of yin and yang characteristics it mirrors, much like a lock and key. Thus, a more yang antigen attracts a more yin antibody, while a more yin antigen elicits an active response from a more yang antibody.

In the confrontational language of the modern viewpoint, which tends to see the environment as a perennial source of potential threats, the lymphocyte's generation of antigen-specific antibodies is regarded in military terms: antibodies are launched like missiles to destroy their specific target invaders. In the eyes of nature, however, this process is not at all warlike, but is natural, benign and beautifully orderly; the environment's expression (as an antigen) and our complementary expression (as an antibody) harmonize perfectly together, and the natural result is peace, or biochemical neutrality.

What makes the antibody and sensitized lymphocytes so "smart"? To begin with, all of our cells and molecules may be said to contain a high degree of intelligence. This is shown collectively by the three primary attributes of the immune system: *specificity*, *recognition*, and *memory*. Immunologic specificity is of a very high order and is dependent on the recognition mechanism used by antibodies to identify complementary antigens. With very high specificity, the antibody binds to only one antigen, whereas with less specificity the antibody binds to two or more antigens. Recognition occurs on two levels: in addition to recognizing compatible binding partners (antigens), antibodies are essentially able to discriminate at a very high level between one's own and very similar but foreign molecules. Thus it is highly rare for antibodies to be made to one's own body proteins, even when these same proteins may be very antigenic in other individuals. A lymphocyte can therefore recognize what is "self" and what is "non-self." Memory gives the immune cells and antibodies the ability to respond when the antigen is introduced a second time. These three characteristics of immunologic intelligence are interdependent, and the degeneration or lack of any one would lead to the malfunctioning of the immune system as a whole.

In allergy, the body's intelligence becomes distorted, and it no longer can discriminate and quietly neutralize normally harmless substances introduced by the environment. What is called an antigen for a healthy person is called an allergen for an allergic person; in other words, it is the person's response, not any intrusive quality of the antigen, that defines it as an allergen. Upon second exposure, the allergen enters the body and elicits the formation of the primary allergy antibody, called *immunoglobulin E* (IgE). The antibodies then tend to collect in a particular organ or tissue of the body which will mark the site of the initial allergic symptoms. Since the blood carries substances throughout the entire body, antibodies can travel to any area—but preferably where there are mucus deposits—to set the stage for an allergic reaction. For instance, asthmatic symptoms occur because of an antigen-antibody reaction in the bronchial tubes of the lungs. Hay fever symptoms result from the reaction occurring in the nasal mucosa. Food allergy initially involves a reaction in the intestines. Reactions in the skin manifest in rashes or hives. The IgE antibodies attach to certain immunologic cells called *mast cells*, which are present in the various shock organs—the lungs, intestines, nose, and skin. The mast cell, having been "sensitized" by repeated exposure to the antibody-allergen complex, releases histamine or histamine-like chemical substances. These substances will circulate through the body and affect the shock organ by producing some visible alteration of the tissue. For example, there may be spasms of smooth muscles encircling the bronchial tubes in the case of asthma; or dilation of blood vessels as occurs in the nose with hay fever; or edema (swelling) as seen in hives.

These observations bring us again to a crucial point about antibodies and allergens. The allergens, in themselves, are not abnormal or poisonous. What is abnormal is the increased reactivity of the allergic person to these substances. Rather than seek the problem without, commonsense tells us to look within, to consider the harmony of immune components—the B- and T-cells, the antibodies, the central nervous system, and other parts of our natural protection. It is our own physiological quality, not the environment, which is out of balance.

Microscopic Disharmony

Recent immunological findings regarding the differences in antibodies in allergic people compared to normal people offer some interesting clues to the fundamental nature of these elements and the underlying cause of allergy. It has been established that the IgE antibodies in allergy are biochemically different from the IgE antibodies in normal individuals. These particular antibodies of the IgE class, often called *reagins*, have been shown experimentally to have an unusual affinity for skin and mucus membranes, and tend to attach quickly to basophils and mast cells. Some immunologists have contended that these reagins constitute an "abnormal sub-class" of cell-fixing antibody.

We can also consider the observation which forms the basis for many laboratory tests used to demonstrate the presence of the abnormal antibodies. In non-allergic persons, the union of antigen and antibody produces a visible precipitation or clumping in a previously clear solution. In allergic individuals, the opposite happens. Although the allergic antibodies are still very specific and capable of reacting with their corresponding allergens, they are not capable of producing the clumps or aggregations of antibody-allergen complexes. Instead, the immune complexes remain dispersed or spread out in solution. This indicates that the basic yang, centripetal or gathering tendency of the antibody has been diminished. In other words, there is a prevailing excess of yin centrifugal energy in the allergic individual.

Previously, we distinguished the yin character of the B-cell from the yang character of the T-cell. Allergy is produced by an excessively yin condition, which makes the B-cell itself excessively yin, producing an abnormal quality of antibody, and often an excess of these antibodies. At the same time, the T-cell loses its essential yang quality, and thus the distortion of its important regulatory functions. As a whole, the immune system becomes dominated by the more centrifugal or expansive energy created by the individual's diet and lifestyle.

Modern Views and Approaches

In ancient times, health was equated with living in harmony with nature, eating a simple balanced diet, and living to an active old age. This is actually the meaning of macrobiotics as it was historically expressed in the writings of Hippocrates, Aristotle, Galen, and others. Illness was viewed as a way of balancing or adjusting the body according to the extent of its disharmony with nature. In the modern terms of natural healing, illness represents an interaction between environmental factors and the individual's resistance and/or adaptability. The human body has its own "reasons" for illness: it uses illness as a means of establishing its own internal equilibrium. For example, a runny nose is the body's way of discharging excess fluid and mucus from the respiratory tract, and this process may be enhanced by actions such as coughing or sneezing. The result is the respiratory system's ability to function more smoothly and effectively. In this instance, sneezing and coughing serve as protective functions, helping to rid the airway of excess mucus and trapped debris, such as pollen or dust. A cold is simply how the body cleans itself through the lungs and nose.

Viewed in this way, the majority of illnesses are natural healing processes. Fever, for example, is an important means for the body to kill infection and protect itself. The great alchemist Paracelsus and followers of the empiricist tradition spoke of "cooking out" disease-causing influences. This idea relates to the rise in body temperature in the course of fever. The elevated temperature leads to radical changes in the internal environment which then becomes inhospitable to certain bacteria. Also, with the increase in temperature various defense and eliminative processes proceed at a faster rate, allowing the body to regain a more balanced state. When possible, it is safer not to interfere with such processes. Rather, we should encourage or promote their completion. Of course a high fever can be dangerous and in such cases a doctor should be consulted.

In contrast to the traditional philosophy of natural healing, modern medicine advocates intervention with the body's healing processes. Illness is viewed in terms of a chemical change in the body's tissue, often localized in a particular organ. According to this perspective, treatment can also be chemical, directed to the diseased organ(s), tissues, etc., rather than to the environment which is constantly feeding the disorder. Instead of influencing the deeper, underlying cause, conventional treatments aim at suppressing undesirable symptoms or wiping out superficial causes such as organ dysfunction, antibody-antigen interaction, or inflammatory reactions. In most cases, although the specific symptoms are eliminated, the patient is left both physiologically weakened, and with the mistaken belief that a "cure" has been achieved. As a consequence of halting or interfering with the natural process of healing, and of not treating the real cause of the problem, the symptomatic approach usually leaves people more susceptible to future ailments. Continually preventing the body from discharging harmful excess eventually leads to more violent forms of discharge, or major illnesses.

In regard to specific problems of the immune system, modern medicine has held the germ theory as its central tenet for treatment. According to this theory infectious germs in our environment attack the body. These germs or microbes (bacteria, viruses, or other microorganisms) are judged to be the enemy, posing a constant threat to our health. The modern treatment is to counterattack the germs using drugs as ammunition. Antibiotics were the first chemical weapons in mankind's war with infectious disease. Their excessive and imprudent use, however, has allowed microbes to rearrange their own natural defenses, creating new disease problems for modern medicine. As the microbes continue to reorient themselves, more powerful antibiotics are developed—only to be foiled again by some new bacterial resurgence.

The germ theory is a product of dualistic thinking—a fragmentary or disconnected view of life. To cure the infectious state these "enemies" (the bacteria, etc.), must be removed, sought out and destroyed, or bombarded by powerful chemicals. The dualistic view sees the individual as separated from the environment, and the condition—whether healthy or ill—as separated from the individual himself. The responsibility for health is thus entrusted primarily to medicine, rather than to the individual's reorientation of his own daily way of life. Dualistic thinking divides good from bad, friend from enemy, and health from illness, seeing one as completely desirable and the other as totally undesirable. This divisive mode of thought is intrinsic to all of modern civilization, including education and religion, science and industry, politics and economics, and so forth. As long as our basic point of view is dualistic it is impossible to cure fundamentally any illness, whether cancer, diabetes, arthritis, allergies, or even the common cold. The current mode of taking the offensive, or "attack," stems from our ignorance of the true nature of life and health.

With respect to the germ theory, a more monistic or unified view would examine the question of susceptibility: Why have these bacteria established themselves here, in this particular part of the body, at this time, in this person? First we should understand that many kinds of bacteria live inside our bodies in a *symbiotic*, supporting relationship. Throughout our body tissues, these natural bacteria live as working parts of the integrated metabolic machinery—altering patterns of organic molecules so that they become usable for energy. The microflora of the mammal's intestinal tract are essential for the proper assimilation of nutrients. There are normally more than 15 types of bacteria in a healthy person's mouth. Rather than indicating disease, these bacteria play an important role in the prevention of disease. The maintenance of these normal flora is an integral aspect of our natural immunity. If we kill off any of these flora—for example, by indiscriminate practice of excessive radiation of the skin—we increase the risk of disease.

Certain bacteria are attracted to a healthy person, while other potentially harmful bacteria are not; and this attraction is determined by our quality of blood. If our blood quality is weak or deteriorating the germs are attracted to us and can be damaging. Clean, slightly alkaline blood, which creates the foundation for a healthy mind and body, is more unattractive to these germs. It is ourselves that are resistant to undesirable or harmful disturbances, and that at the same time are attractive to the more essential factors which allow us to maintain healthy biological functions.

The science of allergy has adhered to the same fragmentary line of logic which espoused the germ theory. To simplify the analogy we may substitute the term allergen for germ as the presumed causal agent. An *allergen* is a foreign substance which triggers the allergic reaction in allergy-prone people. Conventional medicine considers these allergens to be the cause of allergies, and designs the approach accordingly. The primary approach is avoidance: The susceptible individual seeks living conditions which avoid or minimize contact with the allergen. As soon as the allergen is discovered the doctor or allergist recommends avoiding or modifying various environmental conditions. One may move to a different area or to a special house with a special rug, special walls, etc.,—all of which are aimed at an allergen-free world. In spite of these ingenious efforts, in many cases the allergic reaction persists because some factor is overlooked. Wherever the individual may seek refuge, his susceptibility follows as a quiet companion, eventually becoming loud in the form of some new allergic response.

The next step is to consider some type of "desensitization" therapy, involving injection of a fluid extract of the substance to which one is allergic. The extract consists of a combination of specific allergens and a salt water solution. (Salt is apparently the least allergenic substance to which we are constantly exposed.) For hay fever sufferers, for example, an extract of the whole pollen to which the person is allergic is made. Symptomatic improvement may result after six months to two years of these injections. However, although these shots are sometimes effective against dust, mold, animal danders, and pollen allergy, they seem to have no effect on most food and chemical allergies. This is because food allergies involve, in addition to a basic immunologic sensitivity, some metabolic deficiency or a physiological imbalance of the digestive and excretory systems. The desensitization approach usually offers only temporary relief, and on the average has been demonstrated about 20% effective in treating all forms of allergy.

If the desensitization approach fails the next step is some form of drug therapy. At this point the patient is often advised to see a qualified allergist or a physician who has shown an active, specialized interest in the field of allergy. There are hundreds of allergy drugs on the market today; some are general while others are intended to exert a much more specific effect. The most common drugs used are antihistamines (many different kinds), *ephedrine*, *epinephrine* (adrenaline), *theophylline*, and various steroids. For severe cases of allergy the physician frequently prescribes repeated doses of cortisone, which suppresses practically all allergic symptoms. While drug therapy is generally more successful at relieving symptoms than the desensitization approach, it never treats the underlying allergic disease or cause; and in the process of eliminating the symptom it often weakens the body's natural immunity. Antihistamines, for example, have a neutralizing effect on allergic symptoms such as itching and swelling; but must be taken constantly and tend to make people sleepy. To counter this effect, people resort to *amphetamines*, strong coffee, or other stimulants. And, of course, finding a balance between the two in terms of the proper dosage is quite difficult. Theophylline is a prominent component of most broncho-dilators and has been associated with nausea, diarrhea, vomiting, gastric upset, headaches, irritability, insomnia, muscle twitching, palpitations, circulatory failure, hyperglycemia, and certain kidney disorders. It may also induce toxicity if taken with other drugs, such as ephedrine. Another example is cortisone, an anti-inflammatory steroid which effectively knocks out the body's ability to make antibodies—both allergic and non-allergic. Excessive or prolonged use of cortisone or related drugs has been associated with retention of sodium and loss of potassium, water retention with swelling of the face and body, high blood pressure, psychosis and neurologic disorders, heart problems, gastric ulcers, acne, and the inability to heal wounds adequately. Drug therapies such as these may eventually weaken the body so much that the allergic individual becomes prone to more serious, degenerative illnesses.

The search for a safe and effective medication to treat allergies continues. Most of the research has become increasingly microscopic—from constructing peptides which may block a cell's allergic reactivity site to inserting genes which control inflammatory antibody responses. However, some research has begun to focus on more macroscopic factors such as climate, environment, and emotions. On the whole these are viewed as more secondary, aggravating influences which can make an already (genetically) predisposed person more susceptible to the allergic reaction. This has especially been emphasized with the third component, emotions. One reason that emotional or psychological influences are thought to play such a significant role is the observation of the *placebo* effect. The placebo is an inactive or neutral substance which exerts no direct physiological effect, but may still provide substantial relief as much as 30 percent of the time; evidently, the patients' expectations and faith in the mock treatment are a key element in many healing processes. Some allergists are actively incorporating various "behavior-modification" therapies, such as meditation and relaxation techniques, with an eye on strengthening the patients' attitudes toward healing themselves.

In a similar vein, yoga, dance, biofeedback, martial arts, and visualization have also proven useful. All of these therapies have demonstrated some effect on the autonomic (nonvoluntary) nervous system, often resolving psychic and physical stress and bringing about symptomatic relief. The alternative approaches produce—at least in the long term—more positive results in people than most conventional therapies, because they employ more of the individual's personal resources; they often give the person enough psychological nourishment to create beneficial changes toward a more healthy way of life.

The Nutritional View

Another recent trend in the medical approach has been to consider nutritional imbalances. Ever since Adelle Davis, nutritionists have found allergic individuals to be considerably deficient in many nutrients, particulary the B-vitamins and vitamin C. Although vitamin C in concentrated dosages can provide temporary relief, the B-vitamins have longer lasting effects: because vitamin C is so strongly yin, it merely tranquilizes the allergic condition which is itself yin (yin repels yin). However, the B-vitamins are generally somewhat more yang and therefore more easily balance an overly expanded and stagnated condition, created by excessive consumption of animal foods, refined flour, sugar, and chemicals. These vitamins, of course, are essential to a variety of human biological functions, notably affecting blood cell formation and energy production as well as liver, skin and nervous functions. Four of the B-vitamins, vitamin B_6, vitamin B_{12}, pantothenic acid, and folic acid, have proven experimentally to be helpful in alleviating allergy. These vitamins are essential for efficient operation of the immune system. The most abundant and balanced sources of these and other important allergy-preventing vitamins (e.g., vitamins A, C and E) are whole cereal grains, legumes, nuts, seeds, and green vegetables. Vitamin B_{12} sources include fermented foods (e.g., *miso*, sauerkraut, *tempeh*, pickles, etc.), organic green vegetables, sea vegetables, and fish. (Our daily B_{12} needs are so small that the vegetable sources alone, consumed regularly and moderately, well generally provide sufficient amounts.) When considering vitamin needs we should remember that whole foods contain all that we need, and, taken in moderate quantity, exert none of the harmful toxic effects which result from concentrated vitamin-pill dosages.

Following are some examples of the best sources of vitamins and minerals found in our principal foods.

Vitamins:

A: Green leafy vegetables, dandelion greens, carrots, parsley, kale, lettuce, watercress, spinach.

B_1: Brown rice, beans, soybeans, lentils, kelp, almonds.

B_2: Rice bran, millet, wheat, rye, soybeans, pinto beans, sunflower seeds, sesame seeds, peanuts, greens.

B_3: Whole grains, beans, seeds, greens.

B_6: All whole grains, all beans, rice bran, corn and peanut oils, cabbage, lemons, walnuts.

B_{12}: Fermented foods, sauerkraut, pickles, *miso*, *tempeh*, *tamari*, *natto*, fish, sea vegetables, bran, organic unpeeled vegetables.

C: Parsley, watercress, cabbage, beets, carrot tops, fresh fruits, sprouted grains and beans, squash, green pepper.

D: Dried fish, fish oils, mushrooms, (sunlight is the best source).

E: All whole cereals, rice, beans, nuts, green leafy vegetables.

F: Vegetable oils, olive and sesame oils.

K: Brown rice, green leafy vegetables, cabbage, parsley, (also produced by intestinal flora).

Minerals:

Sodium: Sea vegetables, green leafy vegetables, dried fruits, sea salt, fish, root vegetables.

Potassium: Sea vegetables, soybeans, vegetables, nuts, dried fruit.

Magnesium: Sea vegetables, wheat, oats, rye, soybeans, lentils, green leafy vegetables.

Calcium: Sesame seeds, sea vegetables, green vegetables, watercress, dandelion, nuts, sunflower seeds.

Phosphorus: Cereals, sea vegetables, nuts, beans.

Iron: Brown rice, sea vegetables, sesame seeds, beans, green vegetables.

Iodine: Sea vegetables, dried beans, green vegetables.

Copper: Whole wheat, dried peas and beans, nuts, broccoli, mushrooms, dried currants.

Zinc: Whole grains, nuts, seeds, yellow and green vegetables.

Although the nutritional approach is gradually gaining recognition as part of allergy therapy, the conventional understanding of our dietary needs is still too incomplete to offer a reliable cure. Attempts to determine a link between appropriate nutrition and allergic susceptibility have often been sidetracked by the highly popular study of food and chemical allergy. The prevailing focus is based on the immunological abnormalities in the mechanism of antibody-antigen interaction, rather than on the environmental and physiological circumstances which have created the altered immune responsiveness. To the extent that environmental causes are acknowledged, they are primarily thought to be associated with industrial pollution of our air, water, and food.

Some doctors and researchers, (the "clinical ecologists") believe that our biological foundation is severely declining due to the variety of pollutants generated by our modern industrial technologies. The chemicals now persisting throughout our environment—such as pesticides, herbicides, fertilizers, insecticides, food colorings and thousands of food additives—have surely taken their biological toll. Our entire natural defense systems are going haywire, adjusting abnormally to the many strange, often hidden substances that infiltrate whatever we eat, drink, or breathe. Accordingly, the clinical ecologists recommend whole, unadulterated foods and, occasionally, dietary supplements. Unfortunately, the diets prescribed are generally bland and distasteful since there is little understanding about the proper selection, preparation and combination of natural foods. Moreover, partly because of this limitation, the diets are usually only recommended for as long as a certain food sensitivity persists. When a previously identified food is re-induced with no overt reaction, that food can again be eaten as before. However, sometimes patients may never recover from their hyper-reactivity to many foods, including a wide range of nutritious foods. In this more extreme case, food allergists often recommend a manufactured "allergy diet," a scientifically constructed "allergen-free" conglomeration of essential nutrients and flavorings. This approach represents the general misunderstanding of food allergy, and stems from both an overemphasis on the immunologic mechanism and a lack of comprehension about the regenerative capacity of our daily food. Nature has provided us with an immense variety of wholesome foods from the vegetable kingdom. By carefully selecting and preparing whole cereal grains, vegetables and other natural traditional staple foods, an allergic individual returns to a more harmonious and stable level of natural immunity.

The increasing interest in food allergy represents a significant turning point in medical thought because it has redirected attention to more substantial environmental causes. Still, in terms of healing, food is dealt with as a trigger to be avoided (or suppressed) rather than as the foundation for health or for sickness. This omnipresent fear of superficial causes has paved the way for bizarre drug therapies, highly restrictive diets, and other limited approaches such as behavior modification. The clinical ecologists have branded food allergy as the cause of a host of disorders including schizophrenia, depression, headache, obesity, compulsive eating, alcoholism, insomnia, hypertension, hyperactivity, ulcers, colic, colitis, duodenal ulcers, diarrhea, urinary tract problems (e.g., bed-wetting), arthritis, fluid retention, epilepsy, celiac disease, retardation, autism, gallstones, multiple sclerosis, heart disease, cancer, and others. According to the ecologists, our polluted environment creates an abnormal immune responsiveness (allergy), and food and chemical allergy may constitute the underlying mechanism in any one of these disease states. For example, allergy to either the artificial or the natural ingredients of cigarettes could be the reason why some heavy smokers get lung cancer while most do not. The idea is that continual exposure to an irritant (some chemical) or intense pressure on the immune system could interfere with the body's normal resistance to malignant cells, thereby causing cancer or other degenerative conditions.

The idea that food allergy may be an underlying mechanism for a great many disorders is plausible, but we should take care not to view it as the root of the problem. Food "antigens" are only considered "allergens" because they interact with a system which is already hyperreactive, a condition created by the individual's dietary practices and lifestyle. Until this fundamental relationship is understood and dealt with, the conventional treatment of food allergy will remain unsuccessful.

One of the biggest problems with the modern view toward allergy is the immense technical complexity involved in diagnosis. Sensitivity can involve a variety of factors, many of which are practically impossible to identify. Infinitesimal amounts of chemical gases and dust—or indeed any allergen—can provoke the most violent reactions. And, because conventional treatment involves avoidance of the particular allergen(s), an inconclusive or inaccurate diagnosis will not be followed by an effective treatment. If current trends continue, allergy symptomology may become a field in itself.

The Yin-Yang Balance of T-Cells

Recently, some immunologists have suggested that people with more immediate hypersensitivity may have an "abnormality" or "improper tuning" in their white blood cells. It appears that the T-cells exert their cooperative influence on the B-cells by functioning at times as either "helper" cells or "suppressor" cells. By this theory, the lack of a suppressor cell effect may allow B-cells to produce extra large amounts of the antibodies of the type operating in allergic reactions. On the other hand, when T-cells function as helper cells, they are encouraging allergic antibody production. There are two major questions arising from this explanation:

(1) What makes T-cells function sometimes in a beneficial manner, as "suppressors," and other times detrimentally, as "helpers"?
(2) Why are B-cells, which are triggered by T-cells, producing the strange type and excessive quantity of antibodies in the first place?
In other words, granted that there is a physiological abnormality on the

cellular level, which appears to resonate down to the active protein components (antibodies), what factors create this altered state of reactivity?

These phenomena can be demystified by applying the principle of complementary opposites, yin and yang. When the T-cell acts as a "suppressor," it completely neutralizes the bioelectric charge of the B-cell, and therefore reduces or halts antibody production. The T-suppressor cell is thus more yang relative to the T-helper cell, which has a stimulating effect on the B-cell. The smaller yang charge on the helper cell (relative to the suppressor cell) is not enough to neutralize the strongly yin B-cell, but instead activates it for antibody production. In the overly expanded (yin) condition of allergy, these important polarities are upset, and the essential yang quality of the T-suppressor cell has been reduced. As a result, it can no longer neutralize the B-cell, but instead acts like the helper cell to further stimulate the B-lymphocyte's antibody-producing activity.

These cellular mechanisms are interesting in some respects, but, realistically speaking, they are not practical avenues for treatment. Instead, we must look beyond the biological action of cells and antibodies to the conditions which generate such action. The macrobiotic understanding of biological phenomenon provides a key to unlock these mysteries, and thereby to maintain the future health and happiness of humanity.

Fig. 6. Yin and yang balance of T-cells and B-cells: the normal balance (a) between "helper" and "suppressor" T-cells' effects on B-cells is disrupted when an overly yin condition changes the cells' characteristics (b).

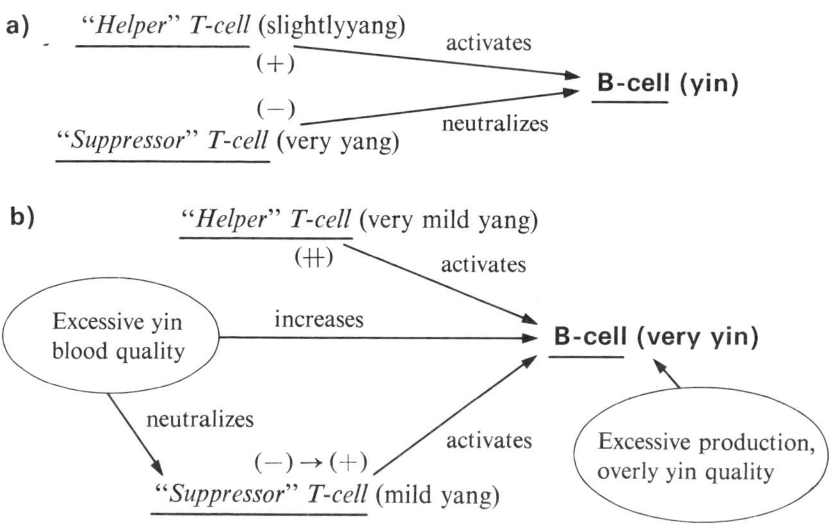

Enlarging Our Perspective

Fundamentally, in order to have a clear understanding of the entire question of immunology and allergy, we have to realize that the modern approach to the problem is inherently flawed—the vocabulary of immunology itself is wrong. The terms antibody and antigen reveal the implicit view of biological antagonism that underlies the modern view, and even the term *immune system* acknowledges the assumption that we are under attack from the environment—for what does "immune" mean if not resistance to destructive force? Such terms, however, are conferring confrontational qualities upon natural phenomena which are themselves not operating by principles of hostility or conflict.

For example, in the case of allergies to cat fur, we have seen that it is the long-term, chronic buildup of mucus and acidic blood quality in the respiratory system that is being discharged through sneezing: if this buildup were permitted to remain in the body's interior, far more serious illnesses could eventually result. Far from being an enemy, the cat, or pollen, or whatever manages to penetrate the barriers of physiological dullness to elicit a cleansing response, are perhaps our greatest friends. If there were an enemy, we would have to say it is our own bloodstream; however, in actuality no enemy exists. Rather, it is simply that we ourselves are not physiologically peaceful or balanced.

A better term than immune system might be *stabilizing*, *harmonizing* or even *peacekeeping* system. Similar systems can be observed operating throughout nature. For example, the Van Allen belts and ozone layer around the Earth serve to balance and neutralize wavelengths of radiation from outside the atmosphere that would be inharmonious with life here on the Earth's surface; similarly, the Earth's oceans and soil serve as gigantic harmonizing or "immune" systems, balancing and effectively neutralizing various environments that arise in excess. It is interesting to note that the type of energy or function classified as "Soil nature energy" in the ancient Chinese system of Five Transformations is also described as "harmonizing," and that the spleen (the center of the lymphatic system) is classified as being of Soil nature quality.

As we saw earlier, the interaction of antigen and antibody is an adaptive act of harmonizing yin and yang. Far from being a hostile process, this constant, natural balancing is vitally necessary for maintaining the strength and stability of the organism. For example, in most inhabited climates we normally need to exert some effort to adapt to changing temperatures throughout the year; this process of constant adaptation keeps our organism strong. Naturally, we protect ourselves against extremes of temperature, just as we avoid ingesting truly dangerous poisons; yet if we eliminate all fluctuations of temperature through central heating and air conditioning, we begin to lose this natural adaptive capacity, and we grow weaker. Adapting ourselves to the changing weather is not an issue of building up immunity to invading forces, but is simply a normal, natural process of adaptation.

By a similar analogy, we normally allow ourselves to be exposed to the differing viewpoints and opinions of others. Just as our bloodstream does not accept everything we ingest (intentionally or unintentionally) as nourishment, we need not accept everyone's viewpoint as part of our own, we digest those opinions, accept some and reject some. Yet we are normally able to respond calmly and intelligently to a wide spectrum of views, and can recognize that even those opinions we ultimately reject are not invading enemies, but are aspects in our environment that are serving to sharpen our critical faculties, strengthen our thinking and keep us flexible.

The immune system is actually a living, biochemical gyroscope, maintaining our physiological balance and stability within a world of splendid diversity. In the sense of the above metaphor, allergies might be viewed as a kind of physiological inflexibility or fanaticism, a state of hampered adaptibility wherein our normal critical faculties are unable to respond calmly to the outside world. In either case, the effort to insulate us from the external stimulus gets us nowhere; but through knowing the keys to changing, harmonizing and balancing our own condition, we can recover our normally healthy capacity to travel freely through our world, enjoying all with whom we come into contact.

3. The Genesis of Allergies

The Immune System of the Fetus and Newborn

Our feeding begins before birth, and actually even before our conception: the quality of the reproductive cells that begin our physical development with fertilization is determined by the food eaten by our parents.

Sperm are created through a yin process in which the cells of the seminiferous tubules in the father's testes differentiate into millions of sperm cells. By contrast, the egg cell is formed by a more yang process of centripetal development or contraction: this can be observed by the manner in which the follicle cells of the ovary arrange themselves in a spirallic pattern with the mature ovum in the center. Therefore, the sperm cell is classified as more yin, while the egg is more yang.

Both these processes of reproductive cell formation are profoundly influenced by the quality of blood and other body fluids, which is in turn created by the parent's daily diet. To promote the optimum quality of egg and sperm, we should naturally eat foods which enhance their production, attraction and reproductive potential. Sperm quality is being transformed dramatically every day by the father's food intake, while the mother's egg quality changes more gradually, over several months. For example, good quality, moderately yang foods such as cooked root vegetables or pressure-cooked whole grains will tend to accentuate the sperm's mobility, while slightly more yin foods, such as lightly steamed leafy vegetables or vegetable soup, will tend to increase egg viability. If however, a man consumes plenty of overly expansive foods, such as ice cream, drugs, alcohol or fruits, he will tend to develop various reproductive problems such as the inability to produce sperm or weak, abnormal sperm. In the case of women, eating from either extreme may also lead to irregularities in the developing ovum, as well as uterine or ovarian abnormalities. The process of fertilization proceeds most smoothly when both egg and sperm are of a strong, balanced quality, creating optimal attraction and strength in the newly conceived child.

Following fertilization, the fertilized egg develops progressively toward the embryonic state in the surrounding fluid of the amnion. After implantation of the fertilized egg in the uterus, the rudiments of all the organ systems begin to develop. The first period of three months forms the structural

---

(For more on the macrobiotic view and approach to infertility and reproductive problems, please refer to *Macrobiotic Pregnancy and Care of the Newborn* and *the Companion Volume: Infertility and Reproductive Disorders*.)

systems, namely the inner digestive and respiratory systems, the outer nervous systems and central circulatory and excretory systems. Organs and glands begin development along these systems during this period. The succeeding period of pregnancy, the second three months, sees the development in the fetus of various auxiliary parts of the body, as well as sex determination, formation of blood cells, and the completion of central regions of the organs.

As the fertilized ovum increases in size, the quality of its nourishment is entirely dependent on the quality of the mother's blood. During this period, it increases approximately three billion times in size, averaging ten million times each day of the nine months of pregnancy. This entire process of development parallels the evolution of life on earth, which is estimated to have started about 3.2 billion years ago. Approximately the first 7/8 of this evolutionary process (2.8 billion years) was spent in water, while about the last 1/8 (0.4 billion years) occurred on land. The first portion, 2.8 billion years, corresponds to the 280 days of pregnancy, and the embryo passes through the equivalent of 10 million years of evolutionary development each day. Embryonic development generally occurs according to the following logarithmic stages:

1. 7 days—implantation
2. 21 days—formation of major bodily systems
3. 63 days—system development; gland and organ formation
4. 189 days—overall strengthening and development

Because of such rapid development, the fetus is highly susceptible to toxins in its body and from its environment. (Adults experience a much more gradual rate of change and can therefore withstand a greater degree of contamination.) For this reason, the mother should exercise great prudence in her dietary practice during pregnancy, and particularly in the first three months (7 days+21 days+63 days). The effects of more extreme foods or substances, such as steak, eggs, sugar, aspirin or sedatives, will usually remain in the mother's body for three or four days. If this is occurring early in pregnancy, the embryo must pass through the equivalent of 30 to 40 million years of some of its most basic evolutionary development in a highly chemicalized or polluted environment. In some cases, this may even result in congenital deformities such as missing limbs or digits, or mental retardation. However, even when there is no evident deformity or abnormality, one effect of an imbalanced, poor quality embryonic environment is that the overall constitutional strength of the newly developing child never receives its full development, creating somewhat more of a susceptibility or tendency toward allergy in the future.

The Role of the Placenta

In the first two months of pregnancy the embryo receives much of its nutrition directly from the mother's *endometrium* (uterine lining). During this time the placenta also begins to provide increasing amounts of nutrition, until it completely substitutes for the endometrium in the third month. The placenta differentiates from embryonic tissues to serve as a membrane at the periphery of the fetus, facing the mother's blood circulation. As a result of various homeostatic mechanisms that maintain the mother's blood composition, a relatively constant concentration of nutrients is presented to the placenta by the maternal circulation. Everything which the mother eats and digests is absorbed either completely or partially by the placenta. The major function of the placenta is twofold: to allow diffusion of foodstuffs from the mother's blood into the fetus' blood and diffusion of excretory products from the fetus back into the mother. The overall integrity of fetal development hinges on the highly developed protective mechanisms of the mother, which come from diet and lifestyle, and are passed on to the placenta.

One of the most significant aspects of the human placenta is its serving as a route of transfer for maternal antibodies. These antibodies have strong protective effects on both the fetus and newborn. In addition to the IgG antibody, several metabolic factors capable of stimulating specific lymphocyte activity are transported across the placenta. Placental transfer also involves large numbers of immunological cells, such as T- and B-lymphocytes. In these three ways specific immune responsiveness is conferred on the newborn infant via the placenta. Most notable is the fact that all of the IgG antibody utilized by the fetus is derived from the mother.

The development of immunologic responsiveness, as determined by the presence of lymphocytes in the fetal thymus, begins at about the end of the third month of pregnancy, between the 10th and 14th week. About the 14th week, lymphocytes with immunological specificity move to the blood and to the peripheral lymphoid tissues of the spleen and liver. However, actual IgM and IgG production does not begin until the fifth month, while IgA synthesis occurs in the seventh month. Even then, the fetus produces only minute amounts of antibodies, unless its environment is stimulated by an influx of antigens from the mother's blood. Therefore, immunity of the fetus and the newborn to illness depends largely on the quality of antibodies that the fetus receives from the mother across the placenta. Most of this transfer from the mother occurs in the third trimester, and involves only IgG. IgA is supplied from mother's milk for breastfed babies, and the other antibodies are also produced following birth.

The mother, the placenta, and the fetus are three intimate and interdependent partners during pregnancy, interacting as a single organism. The unborn baby will receive adequate nourishment and development if the mother's blood is relatively pure. For this, the standard macrobiotic way of eating is essential. If the mother eats in an imbalanced way, a chaotic array of foodstuffs will diffuse across the placenta to cause abnormal fetal development. Substances such as sodium, potassium, and chloride ions diffuse readily from the maternal blood into the fetal blood; therefore, the proportion of these elements in the mother's diet will be reflected in the fetus' blood, and then in the actual development. Likewise, detrimental food constituents such as fatty acids flow easily from mother's blood into the unborn infant's. The placenta has a limited capacity for filtering such unwanted or toxic materials. However, it also serves as a substitute excretory system by selectively and easily passing on waste products such as urea into the maternal bloodstream, to be eliminated by the mother's own excretory system.

As we have seen, much of the newborn's natural immunity depends on the quality of food consumed by the mother. Besides the placenta, two other organs may be viewed as essential filters of the blood which nourishes and develops the unborn baby. These are the two livers involved—maternal and fetal. The mother's liver serves primarily to detoxify blood before it reaches the fetus. Interestingly, the fetal liver serves the same function, since blood of the umbilical cord circulates through this before it enters the general circulation of the infant's body. The constitution of the fetal liver must be strong. Again, this will mostly depend on what the mother ate during the first few months, when the digestive system was being formed. After birth the infant's liver will eliminate the remaining toxic bile over a gradual period of three or four years. This elimination will occur naturally and smoothly if the mother ate well during gestation and if the child is breastfed in the first year of life.

Cow's Milk vs. Mother's Milk

Breastfeeding is essential to the strengthening of the infant's immune system, to its natural immunity, and to proper body growth and development as a whole. Human milk, being of an entirely unique and highly balanced composition, is meant for human babies. Cow's milk is naturally suited for calves. Upon analysis of cow's milk, the amino acids, fatty acids, vitamins and minerals at first appear similar, but are in fact different on two basic counts. First of all, the quantity in which they are present is different. Cow's milk contains about four times as much calcium, three times as much protein, and two-thirds as much carbohydrate as human milk. The different structure and growth rate of calves and human babies account for the varying proportion of these ingredients. For example, at birth the brain and nervous system of the calf is fully developed, and the large amount of calcium and protein is needed to increase its bone structure and muscular development. The human brain, however, is only 23 percent mature at birth, and the nutrients in mother's milk are needed to complete its central nervous system. While the average baby calf puts on 75 pounds in the first six weeks, the human infant gains only a few pounds in the same amount of time. The body of the human is designed to grow more slowly, and human milk serves to mediate this process.

A second fundamental but usually overlooked difference between human milk and cow's milk is size or quality of the molecules. Cow's milk has protein, fat, and various other nutritional factors which may resemble those of human milk. However, cow's milk molecules in general have a larger size than those of human milk. Thus, children who drink cow's milk not only become physically bigger than children who do not, but they also develop more expanded (less compact and generally looser) organs—including the liver, intestines, brain, and other organs. Therefore, emotionally, physically, and mentally they tend to become slow, dull, passive, and dependent. Studies show that people from various ethnic groups who refrain from milk other than mother's milk, for reasons of biological intolerance tend to have higher I. Q.'s than those who do not.

Mother's milk also provides antibodies that deter the growth of undesirable bacteria and viruses, immunize the body against disease and infection (especially against rickettsia, salmonella, polio, influenza, strep, and staph), promote strong white blood cells (T-cells which destroy harmful bacteria), and produce *B. bifidum*, a unique type of healthy bacteria found in the intestines of babies that creates resistance to a variety of microorganisms. In one study of 20,000 infants in the 1930's, 1.5 of every 1,000 breastfed babies died of infant diseases in the first nine months of life, while 85 of every 1,000 fed cow's milk died during a similar period of time.

When infants are fed cow's milk they tend to develop a digestive tract which is biochemically and physiologically similar to a cow's. One study, from the *Lancet* journal of October 7, 1978, reported that such children tend to develop a *rumen* (a stomach compartment found in animals that chew the cud) in the upper end of the small intestine, close to the stomach. The researchers suggest that cow's milk supports massive generation of fermentative bacteria in the calf's rumen as well as in the infant's upper gastrointestinal tract. These bacteria are essential in helping the cow obtain its nutritional needs from vegetable sources. Humans, however, rely on only a relatively few types of bacteria, including the unique immunological type mentioned above. Moreover, human milk is designed to discourage excessive growth of bacteria or foreign microorganisms. The extra bacteria which appear to be introduced and encouraged in the human upper bowel by the consumption of cow's milk eventually reach excessive proportions. These "cow" flora consume nutrients required by the infant and generate toxic substances as well. Under such conditions, the blood quality rapidly deteriorates. The consequence is loss of the immediate protective effect of passive immunity which is normally transferred by human milk, in addition to a limited capacity to develop active immunity.

Another ingredient in milk is *lactose*, a simple sugar that is digested by *lactase*, an enzyme produced in the intestine. In most traditional societies, lactase is no longer produced after the baby is weaned from its mother's milk between ages two and four. As a result, ingestion of dairy products after that age produces indigestion, diarrhea, cramps, and various illnesses including allergy. The condition underlying these disorders is called *lactose intolerance*.

In addition, breastfeeding has many distinct advantages over other types of nourishment, for both infant and mother. Mother's milk is superior to cow's milk in the following ways:

1. Mother's milk contains a smaller percentage of minerals than cow's milk, which is why dairy eaters tend to develop a heavier bone structure and grow quickly. In Japan, where dairy consumption has only recently become commonplace, young children are now outgrowing their parents before completing adolescence.

2. Human milk contains less protein than cow's milk, but this protein exists primarily in the form of soluble *lactalbumin* which is somewhat more digestible than the *casein* found in cow's milk. Casein is relatively insoluble in the human digestive system, it often coagulates in the stomach and produces diarrhea and other digestive disorders.

3. The fat contained in human milk is easier to digest and contains less fatty acid than cow's milk.

4. Due to the unique chemical composition of human milk, the alkaline condition of the body is maintained without the action of buffers. By contrast, regular intake of cow's milk, which is more acid-forming, requires the mobilization of minerals from the bones and teeth to serve as buffers in maintaining an alkaline blood condition.

5. The composition of mother's milk varies during the first few months in order to meet the changing and essential needs of the infant.

Diet and the Newborn's Immune System

Recent research has indicated significant benefits of breastfeeding with regard to the prevention of allergy. Babies who breastfeed from mothers who reduce their consumption of cow's milk will experience a much lower incidence of all allergies than other breastfed babies. This illustrates how the mother's food selection has a direct effect on the infant even after birth, when the infant is still directly dependent on nutrition from the mother. The food ingested by the mother is absorbed into her blood, and this blood is transformed into milk in the mammary glands. The composition and quality of this milk is a result of what the mother has eaten. Even with breastfeeding, unless the mother is eating in a macrobiotic way, the milk produced will be less than ideal for the infant's consumption. This can lead to either an immediate reaction, such as food (usually milk) or chemical allergy, or to susceptibility to other allergies and various illnesses in later life.

In the first few years of life, the infant's various systems, organs and tissues may be modified to a certain degree. The immune system, for example is still in the process of maturation during the first two years. In addition to food, mother's milk provides the antibodies which protect the baby until its own immunological resources have developed. Formation of processed lymphocytes takes place in the thymus and *bursa*, and to some extent in lymphoid tissue of the liver and spleen. During these first years the infant must be provided with a balanced and pure diet. Formula milk or other chemicalized foods will soon overburden the child's channels of discharge to cause weakening in its overall condition. Dairy food actually affects all the organs; however, because it is a product of the mammary gland, it mostly affects human glands and related organs. The most commonly affected, relative to allergies, are the thyroid gland, pituitary gland, spleen and nasal cavities. Many people who eat dairy food have mucus accumulations in the nasal cavities and inner ear, resulting in hay fever and hearing difficulty. Fat and mucus accumulations in the lung air sacs causes breathing capacity to decrease, and a tendency to develop asthma. Accumulation of fatty deposits in the kidneys and gallbladder leads to stones as well as a diminished capacity to eliminate wastes or toxins. Finally, if the infant receives white refined sugar, refined carbohydrates, excessive fruits or juices and food additives in addition to dairy food, its natural immunity will deteriorate rapidly.

It is an intesting fact that among food allergies, the most frequent for infants is allergy to cow's milk. Allergy to human milk exists only in cases where the mother is consuming dairy food during and after pregnancy, as well as artificial foods and sugar. In the beginning, human babies are not attracted to cow's milk, but when it is imposed on them they become accustomed to it. Eventually, as they grow older, they become emotionally attached to cow's milk and continue to consume it regularly. Thus, when people are told that cow's milk is at the root of the allergy problem, many scoff or react defensively. In traditional societies, cow's milk was rarely consumed or was considered more as supplemental food. These people would be appalled at the huge quantities consumed by modern societies. There is also some evidence that traditional societies today have a much lower rate of allergy than those in the milk drinking industrialized world.

Recently, some physicians have recognized dairy food as not simply allergenic, in and of itself, but also as a factor which may be influencing the onset of allergies on a more subtle level. Often referred to as "cow's milk protein," dairy food is now regarded by some as more than just an allergen because of some interesting observations emerging from milk allergy cases. Allergists have noted that milk-sensitive individuals who avoid dairy products for a period of time will often eventually regain their tolerance to these foods, at least to a generally acceptable degree. (This occurs with allergies to other types of food as well.) However, these doctors also occasionally report the disappearance of various other allergies in the course of the milk-free regimen. Furthermore, if tolerance to milk is restored, and the milk is re-introduced, the milk allergy no longer exists, but other allergies—such as *perennial rhinitis* or hay fever—may crop up soon, often within several weeks. For this reason, people with very severe allergies who are beginning the macrobiotic way of eating are advised to take particular care to avoid dairy food. If such food is taken even in small amounts, the immunologic abnormality may easily persist or return, and sneezing, excessive itching, skin rashes, or other allergic symptoms become manifest again within a short time. Our natural immunity is highly sensitive to the combination of cow's milk and sugar so several years of balanced eating and living are usually necessary to completely relieve the tendency.

The dairy-and-sugar combination often provides the foundation for allergy, while other expansive factors—including tropical fruits and fruit juices, soda pop and excessive consumption of liquids, nightshade vegetables, refined flour products, honey, artificial sweeteners and food additives—enhance allergic susceptibility. We may gain insights into the bio-energetic effect of the milk-and-sugar combination by comparing cow's-milk-fed infants and breastfed infants as well as children who drink cow's milk often and children who do not drink cow's milk. From this perspective, we can readily distinguish differences in mentality and intellectuality. The former group tends to be more dull, cloudy, and less intelligent. It is also worth noting that although milk-drinking people are slow, they do have a gentle character—similar to a cow's. However, when these people also consume plenty of white sugar and other refined carbohydrates, their behavior becomes unpredictably violent and hyperreactive. In similar fashion, dairy food confers "dumbness" on the immunologic cells, which is then transformed into hyperreactivity by the addition of sugar, food additives, and other strong yin factors. The disharmonious influence of milk and sugar is therefore twofold: both nervous and immune functions become abnormal. Since these two systems are most vulnerable to imbalanced nutrition in early life, it is probable that most allergy cases originate at this time—even though they may not actually manifest until later in life.

In summary, the natural immunity of the infant, and therefore its resistance to allergy and other disorders, is a result of the mother's eating and daily way of living. The father, too, influences the infant's development, though in a more indirect, psychological way, and can strive to make the mother's circumstances as harmonious and agreeable as possible to support her efforts in maintaining this vital, formative environment. Altogether, the parents' continual reflection on their own diet and way of life can create a child full of vitality and enduring natural physiological stability within his environment.

The Development of Allergy

The macrobiotic view of allergy is based on the understanding of the relation between humanity and the environment; this relationship is similar to that existing between the embryo and placenta. The embryo's entire development is molded by the quality of nourishment and protection furnished by the placenta. If the placenta's quality becomes weakened—as when toxins or fatty acids are passed on from the mother's bloodstream or by various negative psychological influences—the developing fetus is weakened also. In like manner, our larger environment is feeding us all the time through the food we eat and the air we breathe, as well as by non-physicalized, vibrational influences such as light, sound and electromagnetic radiation. If the air, food and water upon which our life depends becomes contaminated, our bodies will eventually begin to degenerate and our natural ability to resist disease is diminshed. By the same analogy, the proper selection and preparation of daily food from the environment around us continues to confer on us the same natural immunity originally built up by a healthy placenta and maternal bloodstream.

Up until the end of the first year of the infant's life, the quality of the digestive tract and of the immune system depends upon the quality of the mother's diet during pregnancy and breastfeeding. Through the course of breastfeeding, the developing infant makes the transition from dependency on the placenta and mother's diet to a more direct interaction with the larger environment.

After the child has begun eating solid foods, usually in the second or third year, the progressive development of allergy may take one of two possible courses. The first is that food allergy may still arise, due to the altered development of the gastrointestinal tract as a result of eating dairy foods, refined carbohydrates, sweets and chemically processed or formula foods. However, if food allergy does not manifest, and the quality of blood and lymph continues to decline, other allergies may eventually arise. It is important to realize that these other manifestations are not directly created by the food. Many people who consume dairy food and sugary foods do not get allergic. The reason is that for allergies to arise, the excessive consumption of these foods must first create stagnation or blockage in some organ or system. People with more yin constitutions (more delicate bone structure, thinner, and taller stature) will often be more readily susceptible to such stagnation. If the bloodstream is filled with fat and mucus, excess will begin to impede the filtering and eliminating activities of the lungs and kidneys. Due to the lack of their cleansing functions, the blood quality continues to deteriorate and the lymphatic system is eventually affected.

General lymphatic troubles are always paralleled by deterioration of blood quality, since some of the fluids and other elements of the blood are constantly being channelled through the lymphatic network to be filtered out and neutralized. Cleansing or filtration is fulfilled by the many tiny bean-shaped glands, or lymph nodes, which contain both lymphocytes and reticuloendothelial cells. These lymph nodes are the primary filters of the blood stream, keeping it free of possibly injurious agents. It these delicate glands become clogged—usually as a result of too much fatty acid in the lymph fluid—a general expansion and inflammation of the lymphatic nodes and organs results. This is caused by overconsumption of refined and artificial foods, milk and dairy products, sugar, soft drinks, tropical fruits and vegetables and other more extreme, acid forming foods. Swollen lymph glands represent a healthy reaction of the body to localize, neutralize and discharge this excess.

When the lymph nodes become clogged or inefficient, or when undesirable material enters the bloodstream directly without traversing the lymphatic system, the spleen and liver act as secondary filters of the bloodstream. The spleen and liver both contain similar meshworks of reticuloendothelial cells which act in a direct cleansing manner on the bloodstream, freeing it of debris, bacteria, parasites, and so forth. The spleen also filters worn-out red blood cells from the lymph and body fluids. The liver and spleen are complementary in both structure and function. The liver is yang (compact) in comparison and functions in coordination with chemical changes in the bloodstream. The more yin (expanded) spleen, located opposite the liver, serves as the central organ of the lymphatic system. The

Fig. 7a. The liver, spleen and intestines all play key roles in the operation of the lymphatic and immune systems.

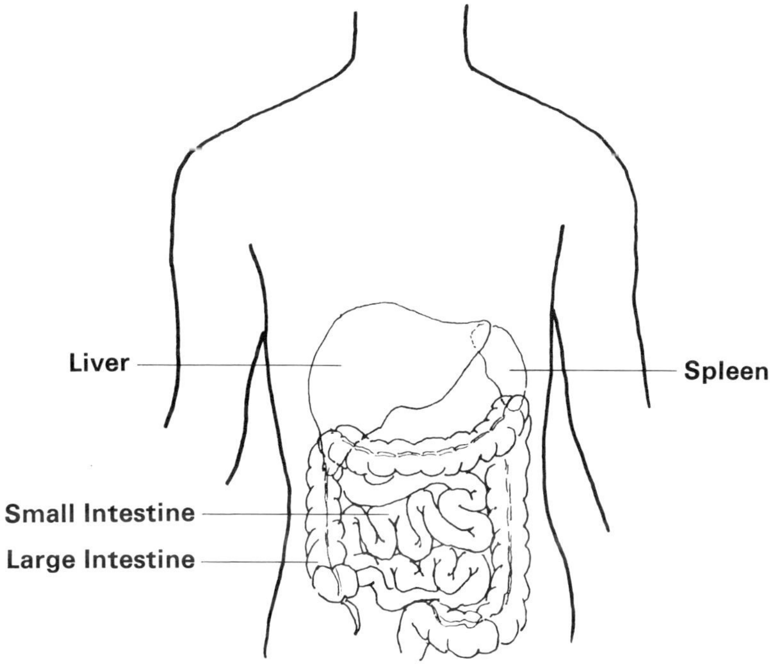

spleen contributes to the formation of white blood cells, especially lymphocytes; stores blood and minerals, particularly iron; produces antibodies; and contributes to the production of bile.

Following the stagnation or diminished functioning of the lymphatic network, the spleen and liver labor collectively to cleanse the bloodstream. If, however, the consumption of dairy and extreme yin foods is continued, a chronic deterioration of the quality of blood and lymph arises, placing an added strain on the already overburdened spleen and liver. These organs, as well as the intestines, gradually become overworked, weakened and exhausted due to excessive uptake of fatty acids, animal protein and chemicals. Since specific immunological cells (B-cells) are first processed by the intestinal tissues, spleen, and liver, the stagnation of these organs affects the production of B-cells. The constant supply of over-acidic and polluted blood to the liver, spleen, and intestines results in an altered quality of B-cells and, consequently, the abnormal antibodies of allergic reactions.

Fig. 7b. The lymphatic system.

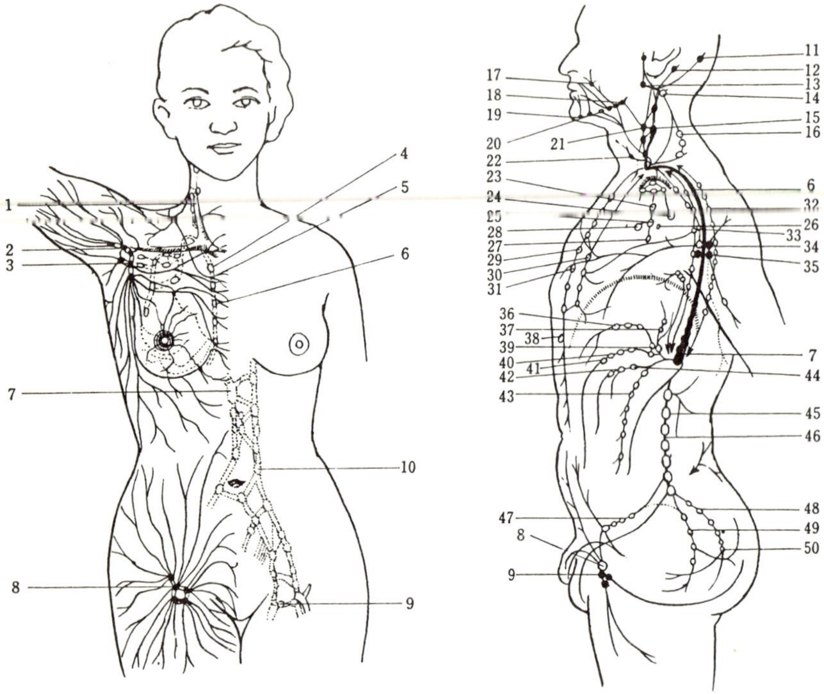

1. The jugular lymphatic trunk
2. The subclavian lymphatic trunk
3. The axillary lymphatic gland
4. The lymphatic trunk
5. The bronchomediastinal lymphatic trunk
6. The thoracic duct
7. The cisterna chyli
8. The superficial subinguinal lymph gland
9. The deep subinguinal lymph gland
10. The iliac lymph gland
11. The occipital lymph gland
12. The retroauricular lymph gland
13. The parotid lymph gland
14. The superior deep cervical lymph gland
15. The superficial cervical lymph gland
16. The inferior deep cervical lymph gland
17. The deep facial lymph gland
18. The submandibular lymph gland
19. The submental lymph gland
20. The lingual lymph gland
21. The retropharyngeal lymph gland
22. The prelaryngeal lymph gland
23. The tracheal lymph gland
24. The pulmonary lymph gland
25. The superior tracheobronchial lymph gland
26. The bronchopulmonary lymph gland
27. The inferior tracheobronchial lymph gland
28. The bronchial lymph gland
29. The sternal lymph gland
30. The anterior mediastinal lymph gland
31. The pectoral lymph gland
32. The intercostal lymph gland
33. The posterior mediastinal lymph gland
34. The left axillary lymph gland
35. The subscapular lymph gland
36. The hepatic lymph gland
37. The pancreaticolienal lymph gland
38. The epigastric lymph gland
39. The coeliac lymph gland
40. The superior gastric lymph gland
41. The inferior gastric lymph gland
42. The mesenteric lymph gland
43. The mesocolic lymph gland
44. The intestinal lymphatic trunk
45. The lumbar lymph gland
46. The lumbar lymphatic trunk
47. The iliac lymph gland
48. The sacral lymph gland
49. The internal iliac lymph gland
50. The anorectal lymph gland

These antibodies will be carried by the blood to areas of stagnation—accumulations of fat and mucus, and acidic blood—where they become attached to mast cells. The end result is highly sensitive areas of the body which may, at any time, given some particular stimulus, set off an allergic reaction. The immune system as a whole loses its essential capacity for recognition, memory and specificity. This constitutes the development of an allergic state.

Nervous and Endocrine Functions

Not all allergies can be related to the interaction between antibody and antigen. By its somewhat broad, original definition, allergy is a state of intolerance and altered reactivity. Many cases of allergy are consequently due to imbalances in the autonomic nervous system.

The autonomic nervous system is divided into two complementary parts, the *sympathetic* or orthosympathetic and *parasympathetic* systems. The orthosympathetic nervous functions are stimulated more by consumption of yang foods such as salt, pork and other red meats, heavily cooked foods, long-term pickled foods, hard cheeses, and strong root vegetables such as burdock or *jinenjo*. Other yang influences include heat, dryness, high pressure and vigorous physical activity. By contrast, the parasympathetic system is stimulated more by yin factors such as sugar, oil, soft drinks, spices, raw foods, cow's milk and soft dairy products, tropical fruits and vegetables, alcohol, and most drugs and food additives. Other yin influences include cold, wetness, light or superficial pressure, synthetics, microwave radiation, and more mental activity or contemplation.

Fig. 8a. The autonomic nervous system.

	Orthosympathetic (▽)	*Parasympathetic* (△)
Iris (yang)	Constriction	Dilation
Pupil (yin)	Dilation	Constriction
Blood Vessel (yang)	Vasoconstriction	Vasodilation
Cardiac Muscles (yang)	Stimulation	Inhibition
Bronchi (yin)	Dilation	Constriction
Digestive tract—wall part (yin)	Relaxation	Constriction
Digestive—sphincter (yang)	Constriction	Relaxation
Uterus—in pregnancy (yang)	Contraction	Inhibition
Hair Follicles	Constriction	(none)

Hyperreactive tendencies often develop when the parasympathetic system has been continually stimulated over an extended period of time. This condition is particularly common following long-term excessive consumption of sugar and other refined carbohydrate foods, ice cream and other creamy dairy products, soda pop, fruit juices, coffee and aromatic teas, spices, food additives, and various drugs or other chemical substances. Autonomic nervous degeneration (often together with atrophy of certain endocrine functions) contributes to an individual's abnormal sensitivity, along with the increased tendency toward the parasympathetic responses of capillary dilation (as in hay fever and hives), bronchi constriction (as in asthma), and intestinal contractions (as in food allergy). Long-term degeneration of this type results in allergies associated with the central nervous system, including cerebral allergy and associated problems; i.e., anxiety,

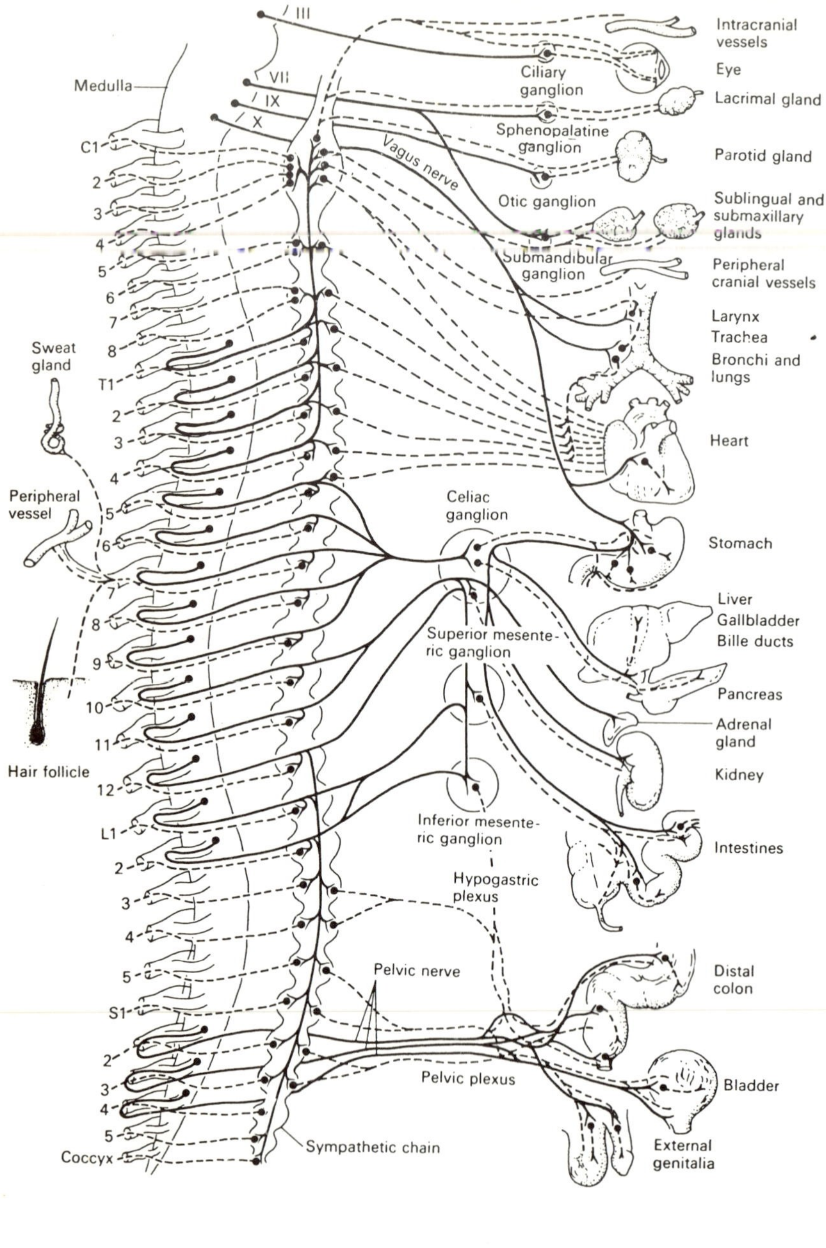

Fig. 8b. The autonomic nervous system.

depression, irritability, schizophrenia, learning disabilities, amnesia and others.

The degeneration described above is often accompanied by a progressive weakening of the *adrenal glands* (part of the hormone-secreting or endocrine system), which are our primary agents for responding to stress. The adrenals respond to various stimuli, both from within and without the body, in much the same way as the autonomic nervous system, by balancing yin and yang directives. While the autonomic nerve fibers send direct signals to different body structures or organs to expand or contract, the adrenal glands effect this communication through the secretion of more yin or more yang hormones, principally *cortisol* (and other cortisone-like hormones), *adrenaline* (epinephrine) and *noradrenaline* (*norepinephrine*). Also, like the autonomic nervous system, the adrenals are highly sensitive to the yin and yang qualities of our food and drink, and are easily disturbed by repeated abuse of extremes such as refined sugar, tropical fruits, heavily salted foods, drugs, heavy animal fat or others. When their functioning becomes chronically imbalanced, we are rendered much more susceptible to everyday stresses such as traffic jams, angry confrontations, rapid temperature changes, and so forth. Overall, such an individual becomes extremely hypersensitive, and often shows a tendency toward epileptic seizures; and this of course may easily contribute towards an allergic state.

Probably most allergic conditions which involve the immune system are accompanied by a weakened parasympathetic nervous system. It is quite common for allergists to attempt to treat an identifiable allergen problem only to find the hyperreactivity still going strong afterwards. In these cases, it is likely that the parasympathetic functions have become abnormally sensitive for the reasons outlined above. These individuals are likely to be "allergic" to such general influences as the cold: lips may swell when ice cream is consumed; hands may puff up when a cold object is held; and hives may appear and consciousness may even be lost while swimming in cold water. In some cases, both sympathetic and parasympathetic functions become abnormal—primarily as a result of excessive amounts of artificial chemicals, dairy and refined foods—so one can also be allergic to excessive heat and dryness. Such people are constantly dreaming of alpine ski trips or Canadian rafting adventures.

Again, the most basic approach to strengthening and balancing the autonomic nervous system and the adrenal glands is to eliminate extremes in our daily eating and return to a more moderate, balanced dietary pattern. In addition, regular activity and a restoration of other more natural daily lifestyle factors is quite helpful; some suggestions for constructive daily living habits are outlined in Chapter 4. In general, striving to minimize our contact with the artificial environment (such as fluorescent lighting, concrete buildings or well-encolosed living spaces with highly artificial temperature controls, synthetic rugs or fabrics, etc.), while maximizing our direct contact with nature, can be a very beneficial addition to the practice of a natural, moderate diet.

Metabolic Problems

Another possible imbalance leading to allergy could be certain metabolic deficiencies. Various enzymes are required in digestion to break down proteins and amino acids; if a particular enzyme is missing, excessive amounts of protein may accumulate to trigger inflammatory reactions and further acidify the blood. Certain foods contain an amino acid which cannot be metabolized by certain individuals. For example, chocolate, various cheeses, certain broad beans, and Italian red wine contain an amino acid called tyramine. When an individual lacks the enzyme that helps digest this amino acid, it accumulates in the bloodstream, eventually causing the blood vessels of the head to contract. This produces the sensation of migraine headache immediately after consuming those foods.

Lactase deficiency is another example of a metabolic basis for hypersensitivity. Lactase is an enzyme needed for breaking down a simple milk sugar called lactose. While more rare among Europeans and Americans, total lactase deficiency is relatively common among Black people, Japanese and Southeast Asian people. However, most Caucasian individuals begin to lose their lactase synthesizing ability at around the age of 13 or 14 years, and many cases of milk allergy in white adults also involve some degree of lactase deficiency.

The Central Role of the Intestines

Physiologically speaking, the origin of allergy is the gastrointestinal tract, the area responsible for direct absorption of food. Digestion depends on a variety of physical factors, such as the number and quality of bacteria, enzymes and quality of tissues. All of these and other relevant factors are ultimately derived from our daily food. Thus digestion is two-faced: we depend on proper digestion to receive the food, and we depend on the food for proper digestion. The small intestine, which may be viewed as the focal point of allergy, is the primary area of absorptive activity. In the course of allergy the primary food to negatively affect this organ is dairy food and oily or greasy food, with refined foods (flour, white rice, etc.), sugar, meat, and chemically processed food exerting a more secondary in-influence. Dairy foods and other oily, fatty foods effectively coat the intestinal villi with fat and mucus (creating bacterial colonies which are quite similar to those in a cow's rumen). The combined effect of these two factors is an altered digestive capacity. Also, while the abnormal bacterial environment created by this condition may interfere with the absorption of beneficial nutrients, it is indifferent to ingested food additives or other chemicals. These artificial toxic substances influence lymphoid activity in the intestines, and are then passed to the liver, which eventually becomes overworked and unable to fulfill its functions of detoxification, the formation of B-cells and antibodies and others. Since the intestines are the origin of many B-cells, the deterioration of digestive functions, combined with stagnation of the lymphatic system, lays the foundation for allergic tendencies.

The Effect of Surgery

The healthy body is always working to clean itself. This involves strong natural immunity provided by an active lymph system and well functioning organs, particularly the liver, kidneys, lungs, and intestines. In addition to the spleen, the lymphatic system relies on the complete functioning of all its nodes or glands, including the tonsils. The main function of the tonsils is to localize various types of toxic excess for discharging from the body. For example, after consuming an excessive volume of sugar, oil, fats, fruits, soft drinks, salads, juices, refined flour, or chemicals, additional white blood cells are created in the tonsils to neutralize any harmful bacteria that may form in the lymph, while minerals start to gather in this region as a buffer for the discharge of acids. In the meantime the tonsils may become inflamed and the body temperature may rise. To suppress these symptoms medical doctors give antibiotics and often remove the tonsils. This causes the fever and inflammation to disappear, but the toxic bodily fluids will continue to circulate throughout the system, and the remaining lymphatic organs will have to work much harder to perform the cleaning and discharge function of the tonsils. The net result is a reduction in the ability of the lymphatic system to efficiently rid the body of toxic excess. The practice of tonsillectomies has recently been linked with a higher incidence of colds, multiple sclerosis, lymph cancer and other lymphatic disorders.

The intestines are generally not considered to play an important part in in lymphatic problems. However, many of the body's circulating lymphocytes are processed in this area, which includes the appendix. The appendix also serves a vital energetic factor in the lower body: The hollow, expanded structure of the small and large intestines is counter balanced by the compact appendix. The intestines, then, are, in a dynamic sense, "held together" by the appendix, in the way a fan is bound together in the center. If we suddenly remove the fan's central binding, it will collapse. In the same way, removal of the appendix (*appendectomy*) causes the intestines to become loose and very weak. This contributes to the possibility of a variety of intestinal disorders such as hernia, indigestion or bulging intestines, as well as the development of a wide spectrum of lymphatic problems. Therefore, the loss of the appendix not only means the loss of its role as a B-cell processor, but also the energetic weakening of intestinal lymphoid activities as a whole. Appendicitis is caused primarily by the overconsumption of animal foods, such as dairy particularly cheese, eggs, and saturated animal fat. This is common in vegetarians who at some point often begin consuming large quantities of dairy foods.

Psychological Influences

The basis for some cases of allergy, particularly those which seem to spring up in the absence of an environmental trigger, relates more to one's psychological and energetic make-up than to one's physical condition per se. These persons may often speak of feeling inhibited in their daily activities by invisible influences, or may describe sensations of some "presence" in a completely vacant room. At times this more psychic disturbance includes strong detachment from or lack of relationship with one's immediate circumstances. Since their character and way of expression are inconsistent, these people are usually labeled by psychiatrists as schizophrenic or mentally ill.

Due to the nature of this imbalance, such individuals demand very careful attention. Although they appear to be very inquisitive, they generally tend to disregard suggestions for relieving their hypersensitivity, or otherwise consider it impossible to change their way of life. For example, when they are advised to try a certain food for their health, they may insist that the food will give them a reaction, even though they have never actually tried it; or they stubbornly, resentfully refuse to eat the food for no logical reason at all. Consequently, they maintain their former dietary patterns, which usually include a large proportion of mucus-producing foods, such as dairy products, flour products, and various oily or greasy foods. In this way they continue to perpetuate their allergic tendencies in a seemingly uncontrollable way.

Scientists in China, Japan, England, and other countries have begun to explore the relationship between electromagnetic fields and biological systems. Kirlian photography has revealed the existence of energy field lines, or layers, around all living things, and some individuals are able to perceive the "aura," an ethereal body of extremely high-frequency electromagnetic energy, around other human beings. These fields are constantly changing through interactions with other energy fields. However, the nature of an individual's field depends not so much on interchanges with other fields as on the individual's biological condition. When someone is healthy, the field around him is very strong, and his resistance to disharmonious energies is likewise very stable. He tends to emanate positive influences wherever he goes. This can be seen when a healthy, vibrant person begins to mingle with a dull or melancholy group of people. The healthy person's vibration often transforms the vibration of people around him, making them more positive or cheery.

On the other hand, unhealthy people tend to create weak or abnormally sensitive energy fields, which leaves them more vulnerable to the negative influences of other disharmonious or distorted fields. For this reason, such individuals may find themselves highly reactive in the company of certain people—even though they may never actually make physical contact with these people. This more complex type of hypersensitive individual should therefore seek the companionship of healthy people as much as possible. In addition, certain types of darker, more humid, heavy or stagnant environments tend to harbor such disharmonious energies more easily, and are therefore less ideal places for these individuals to frequent.

Above and beyond this more specific type of psychological or energetic problem, there usually exist certain more general psychological tendencies that go hand in hand with allergies. The reason for this parallelism is that the body and mind, while usually considered as belonging to two largely separate spheres of activity, are in reality simply two sides of the same coin: they are both nourished by the same blood quality, and both influenced by the same environmental conditions. Consequently, any condition arising in the body will inevitably show itself in the activities of the mind as well, and vice versa.

In particular, a person with allergies often exhibits a certain mental inflexibility, commonly appearing as a lack of the ability or willingness to listen openly to new viewpoints or tolerate certain types of people or situations. Since most allergic conditions involve a strong component of excessive yin factors, some more yin character traits (such as openness, friendliness, gentleness or an easygoing nature) are often exhibited on the surface; but when certain specific topics or situations are touched upon, the more unbending attributes of psychological intolerance may suddenly appear, even bordering on extreme stubbornness or fanaticism.

With the change of physiological condition brought about by a more balanced, moderate way of eating, these more extreme character traits also tend to automatically dissolve. At the same time, it is helpful to approach the entire situation from both sides at once; in other words, striving to achieve a more tolerant, flexibly adaptive and moderate state of mind can in turn positively influence the person's recovery from the physiological allergic condition.

The Dual Nature of Allergy

As outlined in Chapter 1, the development of sickness can be understood in terms of seven stages, the first four constituting sicknesses of adjustment and the last three constituting degenerative illnesses. Allergy may be classified as both an adjustment and a degenerative illness. By considering the mechanism of the allergic reaction and its cellular effects we can see how it contains both positive and negative aspects.

Allergy is characterized by the overexpanded, loose condition of organs and tissues—particularly those involved with digestion and immunity. A mechanism which might be considered positive or adaptive would balance this overly yin state—through contraction. During an allergic reaction, cells located in and around mucus accumulations are stimulated by the allergen-antibody combination to release a wondrous assortment of chemicals (histamine, bradychinin, and a number of other natural chemicals). These substances provide several essential physiological functions: increasing the flow of fluids in and out of blood vessels; influencing the amount and type of fluid produced by mucus glands; and making the muscles and tissues of the internal organs contract. In addition, the functions of the autonomic nervous system, the adrenal glands and other actions of the body supports this compensating ability. All of these effects serve to relieve the overly expanded, loose, or watery condition which is characteristic of allergy-prone people. During healthy, normal functioning, these balancing chemicals are being released constantly in moderate quantities to regulate our natural biologic processes, including the temporary abatement of excess body fluids and expanded tissues. However, in the allergic individual, these substances literally explode from the mast cells to counter the excessively expanded state. The result is temporary tightening relief to the afflicted organs and the increased possibility for discharge of excess fluids, as demonstrated by a hay fever nasal discharge or skin allergies such as hives and eczema. In this sense, allergy is simply the body's exaggerated expression of adjustment to a highly imbalanced internal environment.

Unfortunately, allergy is a far cry from simple adjustment. Its more negative or maladaptive side lies in some of the other effects of the allergen-antibody reaction which underlie physical discomfort. As the blood becomes continually acidic over short periods of time—following repeated consumption of an imbalanced diet—the body cells themselves begin to accumulate acid (hydrogen ions). This highly acidic fluid causes the cells in areas of allergic reactions—these located in or around mucus deposits—to become more expanded and fragile. During an allergic reaction, the affected cells discharge hydrogen ions, making the extracellular fluid highly acidic (*acidosis*). As allergens also trigger the release of histamine and other substances which increase cell permeability, the acidic fluid spreads rapidly to other areas of the body, causing irritation to other tissues, organs and systems. The increase and accumulation of such fluid in a particular part of the body produces swelling or *edema* and its accompanying discomfort. Also, various organs, including the brain, can pick up this acidic fluid, producing inflammation and/or pain in these areas.

In other words, the exaggerated, overly yin condition which underlies allergy evokes a similarly exaggerated, overly yang physiological gesture; and the result is not harmony but a disturbing uncomfortable and at times even life-threatening juxaposition of extremes. Accordingly, one cannot approach the overly yin condition of, for example, asthma by simplistically deciding to avoid eating or drinking anything yin and consuming a strongly yang diet. While this step would quickly begin to neutralize the underlying more yin condition, it would likely serve to aggravate the tendency toward more yang, compensating attacks. In the case of asthma, for example, though the dietary guidelines suggested in Chapter 5 (in the section on asthma) are slightly more yang (to balance the underlying condition), this is meant to be only a mild emphasis; and the type of preparation suggested for use in the case of an asthma attack, *kuzu* sweetened with barley malt, is slightly on the yin side.

In other words, it is impractical and ineffective to adopt a one-sided approach; instead, by avoiding the more extreme foods (listed in the next chapter) and relying for a period of several months on a very well balanced variety of whole, natural foods with slightly more yang but generally balanced qualities, the excessive conditions and reactions of allergy can be modified and gradually dissolved, and the complementary yin and yang functioning of the lymphocyte, autonomic nerve, adrenal hormone and other balancing systems can be built up, leading to a state of overall physiological integrity. These physical changes are reflected in the more happy, positive and outgoing expression that characterizes healthy human beings, and we soon come to realize that the genuine expression of our humanness is one of profound health, happiness and freedom from artificial limitation.

4. The Macrobiotic Approach to Allergies

The following guidelines represent a standard or average macrobiotic way of eating, and can be safely followed by anyone already in generally good health to avoid the risk of developing allergies or any of the many other ills prevalent in modern life. At the same time, it should be remembered that there is no one diet that is perfect for everyone. In fact, this general pattern should be freely varied and adjusted to suit variations in climate, season, past eating habits, one's individual condition and other factors. The companion volume *Allergies* in the Food and Cooking Series discusses these and other practical issues in greater length, and is recommended for anyone wishing to follow the approach outlined here.

These guidelines are followed by a section on how to make general dietary adjustments to suit the needs of people with an already developed allergic condition. In this case (as for anyone seeking to relieve a particular health condition through macrobiotics) it is recommended that these guidelines be followed under the supervision of a qualified macrobiotic counselor, as well as an appropriate medical or nutritional health professional. It is also strongly suggested that the reader pursue a more complete and practical understanding of these guidelines by attending qualified macrobiotic cooking courses. A list of appropriate resources appears in the Appendix.

Fig. 9. The standard macrobiotic diet.

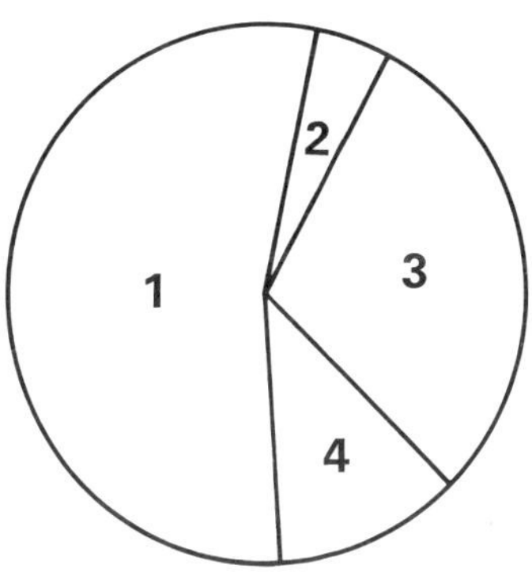

1. 50–60% whole unrefined cereal grains.
2. 5% naturally seasoned soups.
3. 25–30% fresh vegetables.
4. 10–15% beans, sea vegetables and supplementary foods. Plus appropriate volumes of mild beverages.

These guidelines are presented in terms of percent of total daily volume eaten. It is not necessary to weigh or measure precisely the quantity of each food or portion; an approximate comparison of serving size is sufficient. Whole grains can be the principal dish (at least 50 percent) at each meal, with vegetables as the primary side dish, though it is not necessary to include all side dish categories (soup, beans, etc.) at each meal. The total volume eaten may vary considerably from person to person and from day to day, and need not be fixed; but the proper relative proportions of different food categories, regardless of total volume, may be generally maintained.

Whole Grains: At least one half (50 to 60 percent) of daily food may be cooked whole grains and their products. The majority of grains may be eaten in whole form, with a lesser amount consumed as flour, cracked or otherwise processed grains. Grains may be cooked 45–55 minutes and seasoned with a pinch of natural (unrefined) sea salt; brown rice and other whole grains are best prepared in a stainless steel or enamel/steel pressure-cooker. *Grains for daily or regular use* include: brown rice (short or medium grain); barley; millet; whole oats; whole wheat berries; whole rye; whole corn; buckwheat; Job's Tears ("pearl barley" or *hato mugi*). *Grains for occasional use* include: sweet brown rice and *mochi* (pounded sweet brown rice dumpling); long grain brown rice; whole-grain noodles such as *udon* (Japanese whole-wheat noodles), *soba* (buckwheat noodles) and whole wheat pasta; unleavened or natural sourdough whole wheat or rye bread, traditionally prepared flat breads, *tortillas* or *chapati*; bulgur, cracked wheat and cracked rye; steel-cut ("Scotch") or rolled oats; corn grits and meal; couscous; *seitan* (wheat gluten cutlet) or *fu* (puffed wheat gluten).

Soups: One or two cups or bowls of soup (about 5 percent of total volume) may be consumed daily; these may contain a variety of ingredients, including seasonal vegetables, sea vegetables (particularly *kombu* or *wakame*), and occasionally grains or beans, and should be mildly seasoned with naturally processed *miso* or *tamari* soy sauce (also known as *shoyu*). Barley (*mugi*) miso, soybean (*hatcho*) *miso* and brown rice (*genmai*) miso are the most suitable varieties for daily use.

Vegetables: Approximately one quarter to one-third of each meal may include fresh vegetables prepared in a variety of ways, including steaming, boiling, simmering, sautéing and others, including both dishes cooked a shorter time (from 3 to 15 minutes) and with a fresher taste, and dishes cooked a longer time (15 to 45 minutes) and with a heartier taste. The proportion of these two general styles can be varied with the season and climate, the fresher dishes being especially suited to hotter environments and the heartier dishes being more suitable for colder environments. In addition, up to one third of vegetable dishes may be eaten as parboiled, pressed or raw salads and as unspiced natural pickles. *Vegetables for daily or regular use* include:

1. Root and stem vegetables: burdock, carrot, *daikon* (long white) radish (fresh and dried), dandelion root, lotus root (fresh and dried), onion, parsnip, radish, rutabaga, salsify, turnip.

2. Ground vegetables: cauliflower, hard squashes (acron, buttercup, butternut, hubbard, etc.), pumpkin and Hokkaido pumpkin.

3. Green and white leafy vegetables: broccoli, Brussels sprouts, bok choy, green cabbage, carrot tops, Chinese cabbage, chives, collard greens, *daikon* greens, dandelion greens, kale, leeks, mustard greens, *nappa*, parsley, scallion, turnip greens, watercress.

Vegetables for occasional use include: celery, cucumber, endive, escarole, fresh beans (string beans, snap beans, wax or yellow beans, etc.), green peas, Chinese snow peas, *jinenjo* (mountain yam), kohlrabi, lettuce, mushrooms, *shiitake* mushrooms, red cabbage, soft squashes (patty pan, summer squash and zucchini), Swiss chard.

Beans and Sea Vegetables: About 5 to 10 percent of daily food may include cooked beans and bean products as an additional protein source, and a smaller quantity of cooked sea vegetables as an additional source of minerals and vitamins. This may amount to one moderate serving of beans daily or often, and up to several tablespoons of sea vegetables daily. Beans are best well-cooked and seasoned moderately with sea salt, *miso* or *tamari* soy sauce. Sea vegetables may be used as ingredients in other dishes (such as soups, beans or vegetables dishes), as table condiments, or several times per week as side dishes, seasoned moderately with *tamari* soy sauce and/or a mild grain vinegar such as brown rice vinegar. *Beans for daily or regular use* include: *azuki* (small red) beans, brown lentils, chick peas (garbanzo beans); soybean products such as *tofu* (fresh or dried), *tempeh* or *natto* may also be included on a regular basis. *Beans for occasional use* include: black-eyed peas, black (turtle) beans, black soybeans, great northern beans, kidney beans, lima beans, navy beans, split peas and whole dried peas.

All edible sea vegetables are suitable for *daily or regular use*, including: agar-agar or *kanten* (as a gelatin for molds), *arame* (as a side dish), dulse, *hijiki* (as a side dish), Irish moss, *kombu* (for soup stocks, with beans or vegetable dishes, as condiment), *mekabu* (as a side dish) *nori* (as a garnish, condiment or as a wrapping over rice balls or *sushi*), *wakame* (as a side dish, in soups or as condiment).

Supplementary Foods: *Seafood.* Depending upon your condition and desire, you may include a moderate volume of white-meat, non-fatty fish up to several times per week, preferably prepared without oil (broiled, boiled, steamed or as soup) and served together with a larger volume of freshly steamed or boiled leafy vegetables. *Suitable varieties include:* flounder, sole, halibut, cod, schrod, haddock, trout, clams, oysters, scallops, shrimp and others. Whole dried small fish, called *chirimen* or *chuba iriko*, may be used occasionally as a seasoning or condiment.

Seeds and Nuts. A small volume of seeds may be used daily or often, either lightly roasted and seasoned with sea salt or *tamari* and eaten as a snack or used as condiments or in dishes. *Suitable varieties* include: sesame, black sesame, squash, pumpkin, and sunflower. Nuts may be consumed less often as they are higher in oil and more difficult to digest; less oily nuts, including almonds, peanuts and walnuts, may be lightly roasted, salted and eaten as a snack occasionally. It is better to avoid more tropical nuts (Brazil, cashew, etc.) and nut butters; sesame *tahini* may be used infrequently as an ingredient in cooking, and roasted sesame butter may be used infrequently as a spread.

Snacks. It is better to eat balanced meals regularly and snack infrequently, as this establishes a stronger condition of the digestive system. However, light snacks may be used occasionally, including: rice cakes, popcorn and other puffed whole grain products; lightly roasted or toasted seeds or nuts (see above); roasted grains or beans; *sushi* (rice rolled with vegetables or pickles and wrapped in *nori*) or rice balls; salads or pickles; dried fruits.

Desserts. Sweet desserts may safely be enjoyed by persons in good health up to three or four times per week; unsweetened cooked fruit desserts or moderately sweetened grain or vegetable desserts are preferable. *Suitable ingredients* include: sweet brown rice; sweet (hard) squashes or pumpkin (other sweet vegetables such as parsnip or onion may also be used); fresh or dried chestnuts; *azuki* beans; couscous; fresh or dried northern or temperate climate fruits; nuts or seeds. *Suitable sweeteners* (when needed) include: *amazake* (fermented sweet rice); rice syrup or barley malt syrup; dried fruits (raisins, currants, dried apples, etc.) or apple juice. *Suitable thickeners* for puddings and fillings include agar-agar (*kanten*) and *kuzu* starch. In general, it is better to limit or avoid the use of sweeteners on breakfast cereals or as a part of the main meal, as this can interfere with good digestion. Also, the use of flour, granola toppings, crusts and other processed grains in desserts is best kept to a minimum.

Beverages: For sound digestion, it is best to avoid drinking during the meal; also, since the macrobiotic way of eating has a somewhat higher water content in most dishes and is very low in animal proteins and fats (which can build to toxic levels in the kidneys), it is generally not necessary to drink excessive quantities; it is also better to avoid iced or cold drinks. Normally, a moderate serving of warm or hot beverage may follow a meal, with additional drinking during the day according to thirst. It is recommended to use unprocessed spring or deep-well water in preparation of all teas and beverages, as well as in cooking in general. *Beverages for daily or regular use* include: *bancha* (twig tea), *kukicha* (stem tea), roasted rice or roasted barley tea; boiled, spring or well water. *Beverages for occasional use* include: cereal grain coffee substitutes, roasted root beverages (dandelion, burdock or chicory "coffees"), *kombu* tea, *umeboshi* tea, *Mu* tea, or other non-aromatic, non-stimulant teas. *Beverages for infrequent use in small amounts* include: *nachi* green tea; green magma; fresh vegetable juices; temperate climate fruit juices (apple juice or cider is preferable, especially heated); naturally processed, high quality beer or rice wine (*sake*).

Cooking Seasonings: In general, all seasonings may be used lightly, and should not obscure the natural taste of the ingredients used. Natural unrefined sea salt, traditionally prepared and aged *shoyu* (soy sauce) and *miso*, and *umeboshi* (dried pickled salt plum) may all be used mildly in cooking.

High quality, mechanically-expelled oils may be used up to two or three times per week in sautéing or frying (preferably just brushing the pan with an oil brush), and more infrequently for deep-frying or in dressings. *Suitable varieties* include: sesame, dark or roasted sesame, squash or pumpkin, corn and mustard seed oil; sunflower, safflower, soy and olive oil may be used more infrequently, while peanut, coconut, palm and other heavier oils may be avoided.

Additional seasonings may be used in moderation to supply various tastes, including a sour taste (rice or other grain vinegar or *umeboshi* vinegar, naturally prepared sauerkraut or its juice), a pungent taste (fresh gingerroot, grated raw *daikon* or radish, chopped scallion or naturally prepared horseradish), or sweet taste (naturally prepared *mirin* sweet rice cooking wine, rice or barley malt syrup.)

Table Condiments: A variety of condiments may be used sparingly but regularly to impart additional nutrients and added flavor to various dishes. These include: baked sea vegetable powder, sea vegetable powder with crushed seeds, *gomashio* (finely ground sea salt mixed with crushed sesame seeds), ground *shiso* leaves, *umeboshi* plum, *tekka* (a traditional salted root vegetable powder), *shio kombu* (kombu stewed with *shoyu*) or *shio nori*, *nori* flakes, and others.

A small volume of naturally pickled vegetables can also be used regularly to accompany a meal; macrobiotic pickles are prepared from a variety of vegetables, particularly *daikon* and other roots, broccoli, cauliflower and other ground vegetables, and more fibrous leafy vegetables such as kale or *daikon* greens, aged in salt or a salt, *shoyu* or *umeboshi* brine or other salt preparation, for from several hours to over a year.

Fresh vegetable garnishes, such as finely chopped scallions, parsley or watercress, may also be used in moderation to enhance the appearance and flavor of various dishes. Grated *daikon*, ginger or horseradish, usually seasoned with a little *shoyu*, are especially helpful for digestion of seafood, *mochi*, fried or deep-fried foods, or other slightly richer or heavier dishes.

The Way of Cooking

The way in which food is prepared has a powerful effect on its nutritional and other properties, and has a direct impact on health. In general, the kitchen should be kept clean, uncluttered and orderly, so that the cook's full attention can be given to proper cooking. Techniques such as stirring, mixing and vegetable cutting may be carried out with calm and orderly motions, and vegetables may be cut or chopped so that each piece is uniform, to ensure even and uniform cooking for each piece. It is preferable for dishes to be prepared fresh daily; leftovers can usually be stored at room temperature and lightly steamed or reheated when eaten. Refrigeration of leftovers may generally be avoided unless necessary, such as in very hot weather.

The use of longer cooking times, more salt and salt seasonings and pressure generally create dishes with a more yang effect, while the use of shorter cooking times, more water and other seasonings such as oil, vinegar or spicey tastes, and less pressure generally produce more yin effects. These two types of effects can be varied, and may be used to balance variations in climate, season and personal need. (For more information on this aspect of cooking, please refer to the companion volume.)

Foods to Limit or Avoid for Better Health

Animal Products:
- Red meat (beef, lamb, pork)
- Poultry
- Wild Game
- Eggs

Dairy Foods:
- Milk (skim milk, buttermilk, etc.)
- Butter
- Cheese
- Yogurt
- Kefir
- Ice cream
- Cream (sour cream, whipped cream, etc.)

Fish:
- Red meat or blue-skinned fish, such as:
- Tuna
- Salmon
- Swordfish
- Bluefish

Sweeteners:
- Sugar (white, raw, brown, turbinado)
- Honey
- Molasses
- Corn syrup
- Date sugar
- Fructose
- Maple Syrup
- Carob
- Saccharine, xylitol and other artificial sweeteners

Fruits:
- Tropical and sub-tropical fruits:
  - bananas
  - grapefruits
  - mangoes
  - oranges
  - papayas
  - avocado
  - figs
  - prunes
  - coconut
  - pineapple
  - kiwi

Processed Foods:
- Instant foods
- Canned foods
- Fronzen foods
- Refined (white) flour and its products
- Polished (white) rice
- Foods processed with:
  - Chemicals
  - Additives
  - Preservatives
  - Stabilizers
  - Emulsifiers
  - Artificial colorings, flavorings
  - Sprayed, dyed foods

Stimulants:
- Spices (cayenne, curry, etc.)
- Herbs
- Vinegar (except natural grain vinegars)
- Coffee
- Commercial and dyed teas
- Stimulating or aromatic teas (mint, rose hips, etc.)
- Ginseng

Fats:
- Lard or shortening
- Margarine
- Processed vegetable oils

Nuts:
- Brazil
- Cashew
- Pistachio
- Hazel

Beverages:
- Artificial beverages, such as: soda, fruit punch, colas, etc.
- Alcoholic beverages

The quality of cookware and stove used also affect the quality of the dishes themselves. It is preferable to use cookware made of traditional materials, such as cast iron, crockware, stoneware, stainless steel, enamel clad steel or iron, glassware, and others; aluminum, teflon coated and other more artificial types of cookware may be avoided. Cooking over gas, wood or coal is preferable to the use of electric stoves, and microwave cooking is best avoided altogether.

The proper way of cooking is so important that the reader is strongly urged to attend qualified courses in macrobiotic cooking and to study independently with macrobiotic cookbooks.

The Way of Eating

In addition to the selection and preparation of the best ingredients, the way of eating itself has a strong impact on health. In general, upsetting, noisy or chaotic circumstances tend to disrupt digestion, and can contribute to a worsening health condition. Please try to eat only when calm, relaxed and unhurried; also, it is best to eat only when hungry.

Proper chewing is also essential for thorough digestion; each mouthful of food can be chewed at least 30 to 50 times, or until it is in liquid form and thoroughly mixed with saliva. Please try to avoid sleeping for three hours after eating, as this causes stagnation and weakness in the intestines.

When soup is part of the meal, it may be consumed as the first dish. Among various side dishes, the more yang, saltier or heavier dishes may be eaten earlier in the meal, with lighter dishes such as salads eaten toward the end of the meal; whole grain dishes may be eaten throughout the meal. A warm or hot beverage may conclude the meal, or be followed by a reasonable portion of dessert if included. Eating foods too far out of this general order can also cause digestion to be disrupted.

Before and after each meal, it is a helpful practice to express your gratitude and appreciation verbally or silently to nature, the universe or God who created the food, and to reflect on the health and happiness it is dedicated to achieving. This acknowledgment may take the form of grace, prayer, song, chanting, a moment of silence or other traditional forms. To deepen your appreciation of the existence and significance of nature and its foods, you may also briefly express your thanks to parents, grandparents and ancestors who nourished us and whose dream we embody, to the vegetables or animals who gave their lives to nourish ours, and to the farmers, shopkeepers, cooks and other participants who contributed their energies in making the food available.

Dietary Adjustments for Allergies

While the general guidelines given above will serve to prevent various disorders from developing, persons already suffering from an allergic condition may need to follow a somewhat more simple approach, choosing those foods more towards the center of the yin-yang scale, for an initial period, in order to experience relief of symptoms and a reversal of the allergic condition. This initial period may be extended, on the average, for about two to three months, during which time the most uncomfortable symptoms will usually diminish or disappear, after which the person may broaden this scope to follow the more general standard macrobiotic approach.

Also, since allergies reflect various imbalances of yin and yang, such as the balance between T-cells, the branches of the autonomic nervous system, and others, and in the body in general, the goal of cooking for relief of allergies is to establish a consistent, balanced stability. It is therefore important that individual dishes and menus as a whole not be one-sided—overly yin or overly yang—but reflect a harmonious balance of both energies. Also, the way of eating and pattern of meals should be regular, consistent and orderly; for example, it is best to avoid periods of long fasting alternating with overly frequent eating or overeating.

In the next chapter, we will present more specific guidelines for certain types of allergies; however, when dealing with miscellaneous allergies or when not sure exactly which set of guidelines fits a certain situation, the following general additional suggestions for helping to overcome allergies may be safely followed.

Grains: Generally, all whole grains may be used, as in the normal standard guidelines, but with particular emphasis on short grain brown rice, with millet as a frequent secondary grain. It is usually best, however, to avoid or minimize even whole grain flour and flour products; in particular, more hard, dry or baked flour products as well as baked or fried flour products (e.g., crackers, pancakes, etc.) are often incompletely digested and may further an aggravated condition of fat and mucous accumulation; buckwheat flour may generally be avoided. If some flour products are strongly desired, the best choices are whole wheat noodles (not buckwheat noodles), *seitan*, *fu*, or occasionally unleavened or sourdough natural whole wheat or whole rye bread. Partially processed grains, such as bulgar wheat or cracked rye, may be used infrequently; rolled or steel cut oats are best avoided during this initial period.

In some cases, wheat, rye, barley or corn may need to be avoided for a short time. Brown rice and millet generally tend to be the most neutral (least reaction-causing) grains; if necessary, these two grains may be used exclusively for a period of several weeks, with the gradual introduction of the other grains as this becomes possible.

Soups: In order to help clean and strengthen the digestive tract and ensure optimum digestion and elimination, having *miso* soup daily, with a bit of *wakame* or *kombu* sea vegetable and several vegetables, is an essential part of the macrobiotic approach to allergies. For this purpose, it is advisable to use *mugi* (barley) *miso* that has been aged in the traditional way for a minimum of two years.

Vegetables: In most cases, it is preferable to take all vegetable side dishes in cooked form rather than raw, as uncooked vegetables tend to place more of a burden on the lower digestive organs. If salad is strongly desired, particularly in warmer weather, a small portion of "boiled salad" (vegetables blanched for just one minute and then cooled to room temperature) may be a more acceptable choice. The use of oil in the cooking of vegetables is best minimized or avoided during the initial period; and those vegetables listed as being for occasional use are better limited, with the greatest emphasis placed on those for regular use.

Different vegetables have different effects on the body's various functions; and in order to ensure the widest range of rejuvenation and reattunement of these body systems, care may be taken to select from a wide variety of vegetables, often varying daily recipes. Harder, more fibrous leafy green vegetables (e.g., kale, broccoli, watercress) may be included daily or often, as well as various root and ground vegetables.

Beans and Bean Products: Beans are both slightly higher in protein and fat, and often slightly more difficult to digest for an already weakened or stagnated digestive system. Therefore, well-cooked bean dishes may be consumed often, even daily if desired, but in smaller volume than in the usual standard macrobiotic approach. *Tofu*, the dried variety being generally preferable here to the fresh, and *tempeh* may both be somewhat limited, and they are best fairly well cooked in combination with sea vegetables or hearty vegetables.

Sea Vegetables: Due to their uniquely powerful ability to restore immune functions, sea vegetables may be consumed daily, though in modest amounts. All edible types are helpful; in addition to the daily *wakame* and *kombu* in *miso* soup and the *kombu* normally found in other vegetable recipes, a side dish of *hijiki* or *arame* may be consumed several times per week, one to two sheets of *nori* per day may be used in seasoning, cooking or simply toasted over a flame and eaten together with the meal. Sea vegetable powders, such as *wakame* or *kombu* powder, may also be used daily as a condiment to other dishes.

Seeds, Nuts, Snacks: Due to their higher fat (oil) content, nuts, nut butters, seed butters (such as *tahini* or sesame butter) and other oily foods may generally be avoided during the initial period. Lightly roasted sesame or pumpkin seeds may be used moderately, such as several teaspoons per day, either with a meal, as a condiment, cooked into another dish, or as a snack. In general, though, in order to give the digestive system the necessary time to fully digest each meal, regular snacking (even on the "healthiest" foods) is better minimized or avoided.

Seafoods: In some cases, it is better to avoid animal food entirely, including all seafood. In some cases, however, and particularly when the allergic person needs additional strength from his food due to a weakened condition, a small volume of white-meat, non-fatty fish may be eaten once or twice per week, preferably cooked or eaten together with plenty of green leafy vegetables.

Desserts: In order to begin reversing the more yin condition underlying most allergies, it is best to avoid or minimize the use of fruits. If a sweet dessert is desired, grain and vegetable desserts may be prepared several times a week; if fruit is strongly desired, a small volume of cooked fruit may be used as a dessert. Fruit juices and uncooked fruits are best avoided during the initial period of two to three months.

Seasonings and Table Condiments: While eating according to these somewhat more simplified guidelines, it is important not to overseason food or to use too much salt or salty tasting preparations, as these will often lead to a stronger craving for sweets, increased intake of liquids or other forms of yin, if taken in excess. Therefore, please use sea salt, *miso*, *tamari* soy sauce, *umeboshi* plum, and all other salt seasonings in moderation. If you begin to experience an increased desire for sweets, fruit, more beverages, fats and oils or other types of more yin food or drink, it is possible you are using a little more salt or salt seasonings than needed. *Pickles* may be included regularly, even daily, as they help to ensure smoother digestion; in general, vegetables pickled for several weeks or longer are preferable to short-term pickles. *Daikon* pickled in a salt-rice bran mixture (*Takuan*) are especially helpful.

Beverages: Those beverages listed as "for daily or regular use" are those recommended during the initial period; liquid consumption may generally be very moderate. During the first several months of eating macrobiotically, stored fluid, sugar and fats may be discharged in the form of more profuse urination, night sweating or other types of liquid discharge; in this case, these symptoms are not necessarily signs of excess fluid consumption, but are often more temporary signs of elimination of past excesses. The most reliable indicator of the proper level of liquid intake is your natural thirst.

Special Needs

It should be emphasized that every person is unique and has individual needs, and because of this it is strongly advisable to work together with a qualified macrobiotic advisor as well as the appropriate health professional when seeking to alleviate health problems. The suggestions given below are not meant to be followed as a prescription, but serve to illustrate some typical approaches that have traditionally been used in conjunction with the general macrobiotic guidelines given above. In the discussion below, all terms and recipes marked with an asterisk (*) are explained in more detail in the companion volume from the *Macrobiotic Food and Cooking Series.*

1. Digestive Problems. In order to relieve allergies, it is especially important to maintain regular, strong digestion and elimination. Make sure to maintain a calm, orderly way of eating, and especially emphasize chewing each bite thoroughly, one hundred times or more, or until each bite of food becomes liquified in your mouth. Also take particular care not to overeat, and to avoid eating for about three hours before sleeping. Everyday, you can scrub your whole body with a dry or hot, damp cotton towel or washcloth. This helps to activate blood and lymph circulation, and will help to maintain good elimination.

Difficulties with digestion often disappear shortly after beginning a macrobiotic way of eating, without any special attention. However, for very weak digestion you may also take one small cup of *ume-sho-kuzu** each day for up to ten days. Vigorous daily walks can also help strengthen absorption and digestion.

If you experience constipation, you can deeply massage your shoulders, legs and bottoms of your feet, trying to make all stiff or tight areas softer and more relaxed. Also, light massage directly over the lower abdomen can help to encourage better bowel elimination. If the constipation persists, you may take a dessert-sized serving of agar-agar,* sweetened with barley malt or rice malt syrup; this should be prepared in the usual manner, but consumed while still warm or hot (before it has gelled). This may be taken once or twice per day for up to three days if necessary.

2. Menstrual and Reproductive Problems. Maintaining regular menstruation is also important in the relief of allergies. In cases where menstruation has previously stopped, periods will usually resume within several months after beginning to eat macrobiotically, though this may in some cases take up to one year. In some cases, women who begin eating macrobiotically experience a temporary cessations of menstrual periods, while the reproductive organs are beginning to turn there energies inward to begin dissolving stagnated accumulations. To aid in dissolving and releasing stagnated animal fat and protein that can cause the reproductive system to become blocked, you can use a *daikon** leaves hip bath, followed by a douche* made with *bancha* tea; this can be used daily or regularly until the period resumes.

In cases where men are experiencing a weakened sexual vitality, you can make sure to take vigorous daily exercise, and use some side dishes daily that include well-cooked root vegetables, such as carrot, burdock, dandelion root or *jinenjo* (mountain yam).

3. Edema. In cases where stagnated lymph fluid has caused swelling or the accumulation of fluid, some of this swelling may be drawn off by applying a hot ginger compress* to the area, followed by a buckwheat plaster.* The buckwheat plaster may be left in place for about a half an hour, and repeated as often as necessary. (It is better not to use this application over skin that is irritated or on the site of an allergic reaction.) In any case of swelling or water retention, care may also be taken that the person is not taking too much salt or salty tasting food. In cases where the kidney function has stagnated, which is often revealed by a pronounced darkness or pooling of fat under the eyes ("eyebags"), a hot ginger compress* may be applied to the kidney (mid-back) region (once or several times over several days, for about 10 to 15 minutes each time).

Respiratory Congestion: Relieving congestion in the lungs or bronchi may be helped by applying a mustard plaster* or hot ginger compress* over the front and back of the lung or upper lung region. Stubborn accumulations in this area or in the nasal or sinus area may also be loosened up by applying a lotus root plaster* over the stagnated region. In the section on asthma in the next chapter, additional suggestions are also given.

Skin Irritation: The section on skin allergies in the next chapter presents some special guidelines for helping to relieve uncomfortable symptoms of skin allergies, which may also be applied in general if temporary irritations of the skin should arise. In either case, special care may be taken not to use artificial cosmetics or skin cleansers, and to keep the area free of direct contact with synthetic fabrics. For washing, a rice bran wash* is a very mild, soothing alternative to commercial skin care products.

The Question of Allergens

The central issue in relieving allergies through macrobiotics is to change the quality of our blood and underlying whole body condition. At the same time, and particularly during the inital period of several months, it may be necessary to make special efforts to avoid coming into contact with the particular environmental factor that has been triggering the allergic reactions. In general, it is especially helpful in the case of allergies to make every practical effort to make your environment as simple and natural as possible, as outlined by the suggestions on daily lifestyle later in this chapter. In the case of food allergies, it may be necessary to avoid certain foods even though they are normally part of the standard macrobiotic approach, such as wheat, soy products or certain vegetables. (This question is discussed again in the next chapter in the section on food allergies.) Depending on the severity of the allergy, the length of time it has been developing, and other individual factors, this abnormal sensitivity will usually disappear in anywhere from several weeks to three or four months, though this may happen much more rapidly in some cases (even taking only several days) or, in rarer cases, as much as six to nine months.

Medications

After adopting a macrobiotic lifestyle and way of eating, it is a common experience for various health conditions to improve to the point where is it possible to discontinue the use of many medications. The question of when or how gradually it is advisable to discontinue medications is a highly individual issue, and is best approached with reasonable caution and in consultation with the appropriate medical professional.

As a general rule, a reliance on drugs or medications should be withdrawn gradually rather than all at once, in stages that follow the gradual change in health and permit a regular reassessment of dosages and their effects. Most prescription and non-prescription medications fall into one of three categories. *Supplements and miscellaneous aids* such as sleeping pills, sedatives, stimulants, painkillers, vitamin and mineral tablets, and others, can usually be discontinued fairly quickly, over a period of ten days to two months. Medicines that *affect or control bodily conditions* include blood pressure medications, diuretics, antibiotics, anticonvulsives, anti-inflammatory drugs such as cortisone, and others. Most medications to control the symptoms of allergic reactions fall into this second category. As the condition in question improves, these can often be withdrawn gradually over a period of about one to four months.

The third category includes medications that *maintain or regulate vital bodily functions*, including hormone supplements or replacements. Mechanical supports would also come under this category, including such devices and procedures as pacemakers, dialysis, insulin pumps and routine catherization. Naturally, treatments in this third category must be approached with the greatest caution and generally take the longest time to withdraw.

In adopting macrobiotic guidelines to help relieve any health condition including allergies, it is vitally important to begin trying to develop, exercise and express your own intuition. As in all areas of life, the appropriate way to eat macrobiotically can never be reduced to set formulas or rigid rules, because each person is a unique, constantly changing manifestation of nature. Initially, as we follow written guidelines or principles learned through cooking classes or cookbooks, macrobiotic cooking often appears to be a technique or science; but as our awareness of the dynamic nature of our health and our food grows, we gradually begin to realize that eating macrobiotically is truly an art.

Guidelines for a Natural Way of Life

In order to establish a firm foundation of natural health, physiological stability and adaptibility, it is of course vital that we recognize those factors in our daily lives that have originally led to our symptoms of suffering or sickness, so that we may seek to correct them. The problem of allergies, while physiological in its mechanisms, is a manifestation of a generally unstable, extreme or disorderly lifestyle, of which imprudent eating and drinking are the central but not the only feature. When we reflect on the way of living that has led to the chronic overreactions of allergies, we can usually discover many ways in which our day to day home environment, behavior and thinking have served to cut us off from the nourishing energies and beneficial features of the world around us.

The following are some simple guidelines for daily living that can help to begin reorienting our condition and our view toward a more healthy, mutually supportive relationship with our daily circumstances, our friends and social environment, and the natural universe itself.

1. Please live each day happily without being preoccupied with your state of health.

2. Include some regular physical exercise in your daily life, including activities such as scrubbing floors, cleaning windows, washing and cleaning your home, carpentry, gardening, or others. Some form of systematic exercise program may be very helpful, such as yoga, *Do-In* (self-masssge and corrective exercises), martial arts, athletics, or even

simply regular long walks. Regular deep breathing exercise can also be very helpful in strengthening the body's discharging of accumulated toxins, as well as calming your mind and establishing a generally more even energy flow.

3. For the deepest and most restful sleep, try to retire before midnight and rise early in the morning. Again, it is advisable to avoid eating for three hours before sleeping.

4. Go outdoors often, and try to walk barefoot on the soil, grass or beach every day. Keep large green plants in your home to enrich the fresh oxygen content of the air, and open windows when possible to permit better circulation of fresh air. It is best to use central heating and air conditioning only to the extent necessary for reasonable comfort; please allow yourself to experience the natural seasonal changes of temperature appropriate to the climate where you live.

5. It is better to avoid lengthy, hot baths or showers, as they can deplete your body of minerals and have a weakening effect. Bathe as needed, but preferably use brief baths or showers with a moderate temperature. If you feel fatigued after bathing, you may drink a small cup of *tamari-bancha** or *miso* soup to replenish your energy.

6. To vitalize your blood and lymph circulation, scrub and massage your whole body with a hot, damp cotton towel or washcloth until your skin becomes red, each morning or night. At the least, scrub the arms, legs, hands and feet, including each finger and toe.

7. All daily living materials should be as natural as possible, as synthetic fabrics and other man-made materials can disrupt the energies you receive from the natural environment. Use cotton clothing directly next to your skin, especially for undergarments; and for the best health, excessive metallic jewelry or accessories on the fingers, neck or wrists should be kept to a minimum. Cotton sheets, towels, blankets and pillowcases, and incandescent lighting, natural wood furnishings and wool or cotton carpeting all contribute to a more natural environment.

8. Avoid or minimize the use of electric appliances close to your body, including electric shavers, hair dryers, blankets, heating pads, toothbrushes, etc. It is especially advisable to use a gas or wood stove for all cooking, rather than electric or microwave devices. It is also preferable to use earthenware, glassware, cast iron or stainless steel cookware

rather than aluminum, teflon coated or electric cooking pots.

9. Television, particularly color television, exerts a draining influence, as do all radiation emitting devices such as computer display terminals, video games and X-ray machinery; if you watch television, do so in moderation and from a reasonable distance, and deep your contact with all such devices to the minimum necessary.

10. To maintain the healthy functioning of your skin, which is a vital part of the excretory system's regular discharging of toxins and excesses, avoid using chemically produced cosmetics and body care products; try to use those natural cosmetics made from vegetable sources only. For care of teeth, use natural toothpaste, sea salt, *dentie** or clay.

The decision to begin establishing a more balancing, health-supporting diet and way of living naturally includes the resolve to adopt a more positive, optimistic and embracing outlook. Seek to live each day happily, without being preoccupied with your condition or dwelling on negative thoughts, ideas or emotions. Remember that the change from sickness to health, or from unhappiness to happiness, rarely proceeds in a straight line: you will likely experience temporary periods of feeling somewhat worse again, together with times of more clear-cut improvement when you feel progressively much better.

This is actually a natural cycle, an example of the universal rhythms of yin and yang which occur everywhere and in everything. During any more difficult periods, it is helpful to read accounts of those whose lives have changed for the better through adopting macrobiotics, such as the experiences of relief of allergies recounted in the last chapter of this book. It is also helpful to renew and deepen your regular contact with nature, and to keep an active exchange with your family and friends, rather than isolating yourself. The following daily practices are also helpful in reorienting your daily life towards a more stable, personally and socially harmonious lifestyle:

1. Greet everyone you meet happily and with appreciation.

2. Initiate and maintain an active, regular correspondence with all family members, often expressing your gratitude for their being a part of your life.

3. Enlarge your circle of friends and acquaintances, including people from all types of circumstances and walks of life.

4. Share your food with others often; food prepared in larger quantities is always more satisfying, and the act of sharing good food is a universal gesture of human brotherhood and sisterhood.

5. Put aside some time daily to make yourself quiet and peaceful, and offer your thanks to your ancestors, teachers and elders, and your dedication to help and support those who look to you for guidance. This may take the form of a simple meditation or prayer, or a simple daily dedication towards the furthering of human peace and happiness.

Harmony through Self-Reflection

As we saw in a previous chapter, our modern, scientific approach to allergies is based on the view of dualism, which separates man from nature, good from bad and friend from enemy. On a physiological level, this kind of dualistic, divisive viewpoint is translated into the extreme hostilities and overreactions of the allergic symptoms, or in the case of auto-immune disorders (which we will look at in the next chapter), as a confusion of self and "enemy." Through the macrobiotic perspective, we saw that what is termed the "immune system," or our "defense" for protection against environmental invaders, might more accurately be termed the "stabilizing" or "balancing" system.

Living in the modern, fast-paced technological world, it is quite easy to come to see ourselves as separate and isolated from the rest of the world, as lone beings struggling for survival in hostile surroundings. But by adopting a more universal, embracing perspective, we begin to see that we are not all separate, but that we are in fact nothing but manifestations of the natural world that has created us and that constantly supplies us with air, sunlight and nourishment. At the same time, we begin to realize that all the influences in our daily lives, even apparent failures, sicknesses, struggles or difficulties, are actually serving to support us and challenge us to strengthen our own capabilities, and our own capacity to harmonize with our surroundings. By appreciating the gift of life in all its dimensions, we increase our faith in the integrity of the universe, and life increasingly becomes a joyful and amusing adventure. Finally, we begin to have the direct awareness that no "enemies" actually exist, and that everything is proceeding in a wonderful harmony, which we can experience as such when we are living in a normal state of natural health.

As a daily practice to help develop and deepen this sort of awareness, we may pursue the following types of self-reflection, which may be included in the form of daily meditation, prayer or quiet contemplation described above:

1. Did I eat today in harmony with my environment, my history and my purpose in life?

2. Did I think of my parents, relatives, friends, teachers and elders with love and respect?

3. Did I happily greet everyone I met today and express an interest in their lives?

4. Did I contemplate the sky, trees, plants and stars, and marvel at the wonders of nature?

5. Did I contemplate the works of art, culture, industry and human ingenuity and endeavor, and marvel at the aspirations of human society?

6. Did I thank everyone and appreciate everything I experienced today?

7. Did I carry out my activities today with faith and commitment, and thereby contribute to the dream of a more peaceful world?

5. Approaching Individual Allergies

1. Hay Fever

When people think of allergies one of the most common images which springs to mind is hay fever. Medically characterized as a form of *allergic rhinitis* (allergy plus inflammation of the nose) this condition is usually accompanied by sneezing, a runny nose, watery eyes, and, in some cases, fever. In hay fever, the nasal mucosa secretes a combination of mucus and a clear, watery fluid; conjunctival irritation leads to watery and itchy eyes; and sometimes there is ear pain along with the sensation of ear pressure. Overall, the afflicted person may experience fatigue, irritability, moodiness, and headaches. Hay fever is marked by recurrence during the pollen seasons, primarily spring and summer. Another form of allergic rhinitis, called *nonseasonal* or *perennial* allergic rhinitis, occurs year-round and bears symptoms identical to hay fever. Whereas hay fever is thought to be caused by pollen, the perennial type is presumably due to other allergens such as foods, dusts, molds, and chemicals.

The term *hay fever* originally described the feverish symptoms experienced during English hay harvests. In those days people thought the hay itself caused the "fever." Eventually, it was learned that the symptoms were actually induced by the pollen of grass or trees. For this reason, to the present day, it is still believed that hay fever is caused by pollen. However, this explanation is shortsighted, and only designates the superficial cause. If pollen were the true cause then everyone would develop hay fever. It is true that certain allergic antibodies (IgE) and allergens (e.g., pollens) interact to elicit the hay fever response; but the real cause is that which leads to the susceptibility to hay fever; an overly yin, sticky blood quality localized in the respiratory tract and mucus membranes.

Several general facts should serve to illuminate the significance of allergic susceptibility in hay fever. First, hay fever sufferers are often allergic not just to one type of pollen, or solely to pollen itself, but also to house dust, molds, and animal dander. Hay fever symptoms reach their zenith in the spring and summer, when pollen is freely circulating in the air; however, during the fall and winter, when the individual is mostly indoors, the symptoms may still persist, albeit at a diminished level of intensity. Therefore, there is an increasing ambiguity about distinguishing seasonal hay fever from perennial rhinitis; it now appears that the latter is an outgrowth of the former. Also, it has been widely observed that hay fever often leads to other allergies such as asthma. Moreover, neither the particular symptoms of hay fever nor allergy to specific allergens (e.g., pollens) is inherited, although allergic rhinitis disorders do tend to occur in certain families. What doctors perceive as "inheritable" is simply the tendency to become allergic.

The hay fever individual, like all allergy-prone people, is faced with an interesting set of decisions when the "causative factors" of his condition are revealed. If, for instance, a man in eastern Oregon is told by his doctor that he is allergic to the pollen of the juniper and cedar trees, then he may consider moving to an area free of these trees. But if this man is a lumberjack, then he may also have to consider changing his occupation, since carrying along allergy drugs in the woods may prove too burdensome or impractical (lumberjacks must be able to maneuver about easily in tight places). More common is the case of a farmer or gardener with a severe allergy to grasses or weeds. These people may be compelled to change both their residence and their occupation if the condition is too inhibitory; and even when such adjustments are made, the relief from symptoms is almost always temporary. Because of their predisposition or susceptibility to allergy they will in all probability develop a new allergic symptom when exposed to a new pollen, dust, or mold. At the extreme, there appears to be no alternative but to live in a completely sterile environment.

As part of their locale, hay fever sufferers must not only ponder the climate and the range of potential allergens, but also the seasons for known allergens. Grass poses as the strongest allergen in the West, and it pollinates during the late spring and early summer months. Ragweed is a common culprit around the end of the summer. Trees may offer action any time from the end of January through June. Weeds and molds are most active from August through October. The fact that the pollen season varies in different regions of the United States and other countries is a disturbing reality to pollen-fearing folk. Is it possible that for most of the 15 million afflicted Americans the months of November and December are the only "safe" months of the year? If this speculation is accurate we might expect hay fever types to savor the more northern latitudes, where snow predominates for much of the year. We would accordingly predict winter activities such as skiing or skating to hold preference over baseball or soccer. However, because most hay fever cases are highly susceptible to upper respiratory infection, these people will also find themselves thwarted by cold weather, when respiratory infections are prevalent.

The macrobiotic approach to hay fever eliminates the need for such restrictions, exclusivity, and social alienation. Our approach instead broadens one's range and scope of life by establishing sound health. Neither drugs nor change of locale is necessary; such methods are based on fear rather than understanding. The macrobiotic approach, to hay fever, by contrast, is simple, practical, and inexpensive.

After beginning to follow the macrobiotic approach relief from hay fever usually begins quickly. Within weeks the usual clear watery discharge becomes more whitish, and eventually it is mostly mucus. Once the respiratory tract—particularly the sinuses—are cleared, the sneezing, sniffling, and irritated eyes subside quickly. There may be occasional reactions now and then for a period of several months to a year, as the body continues to rid itself of excess mucus accumulations. However, all symptoms will eventually clear up if the standard recommendations are followed closely. Daily physical exercise such as walking, jogging, yoga, dance, swimming, or various martial arts can accelerate the relief of hay fever.

Cause: Hay fever results from a long-term consumption of dairy foods, oil, oily and greasy foods, flour products and refined grain products, together with fruits and fruit juices, sugar, sweets, and tropical foods.

Adjustments to the standard macrobiotic approach: For an initial period of several months, the standard macrobiotic dietary approach may be followed with the following additional suggestions:

Flour and baked flour products are best avoided: *seitan*, *fu*, whole wheat noodles and natural rise, unyeasted or sourdough bread may occasionally be eaten in small volume if desired.

Oil in cooking may be minimized or avoided for one or two months; *nuts and nut or seed butters* may be avoided, though lightly roasted seeds may be used moderately.

Beans, particularly *azuki*, lentil and chickpea, may be used regularly, but in small volume. If desired, a small volume of non-fatty, white-meat *fish* may be eaten once or twice per week.

A small volume of cooked or dried, temperate-climate or Northern *fruit* may be used if desired for a sweet taste; if possible, though, all fruits are best minimized, and fruit juices or raw fruits are best avoided. Any macrobiotic vegetables or grain-based sweets may be used moderately.

In addition, for hay fever, regular contact with fresh clean air is important. It is helpful to avoid contact with dusty air. Also, for hay fever and all respiratory allergies, good digestion and regular, smooth elimination are especially important.

2. Asthma

The term *asthma* derives from the Greek meaning "to breathe hard." *Bronchial asthma*, as the term implies, is a disease affecting the bronchial tubes (bronchi) and particularly the smaller branches of the bronchial tree (*bronchioles*). These fine subdivisions of the air passages are lined with mucus-producing cells and tiny, hair-like fibers called *cilia*. The cilia serve a cleansing function by moving mucus from the bronchial tubes through the *trachea* (wind-pipe). Also lining the bronchioles are small strands of circular muscles which, through contraction or expansions, can alter the bronchioles' diameter, thus mediating the air flow to the lungs. The asthmatic reaction may result from either bacterial infection or an allergic condition, or both. Either condition may bring about a spasmodic contraction of the bronchide muscles (*bronchospasm*) and a swelling of the mucus membranes. This, in turn, manifests in great difficulty in breathing. In its most severe form, *status asthmaticus*, the ventilating functions may be so impaired as to cause severe *cyanosis* (a bluish or purplish discoloration of the skin due to insufficient oxygenation of the blood) and even death. Recent estimates count over 9 million asthmatics in the United States.

In the well-known and respected medical text, *Pathologic Basis of Disease* (Robbins & Cotram, 1979), asthma is described as a ". . . particularly distressing disease because those unpredictably attacks of severe dyspnea and wheezing triggered by sudden episodes of bronchospasm." The key word here is "unpredictably." The implication is that the cause is virtually unknown. In some cases, similar to hay fever, the asthmatic attacks are triggered by exposure to an allergen to which the patient has previously been sensitized, but in most cases no clear evidence of an allergic trigger can be found by current medical means.

Medical doctors attempt to classify five types of asthma according to the precipitating factor and the mechanism or immunologic reaction. These five are as follows:

1. *Reaginic* or *atopic* asthma, whereby environmental antigens such as dusts, pollens, animal dander, foods, and virtually any antigen is implicated as an allergic trigger.

2. *Nonreaginic* or *nonatopic* asthma, which is thought to be frequently triggered by respiratory tract infection.

3. *Aspirin-sensitive* asthma, in which patients are highly sensitive to very small doses of aspirin and experience not only asthmatic attacks but also *urticaria* (skin eruption).

Fig. 10. Constriction of the bronchi in asthma.

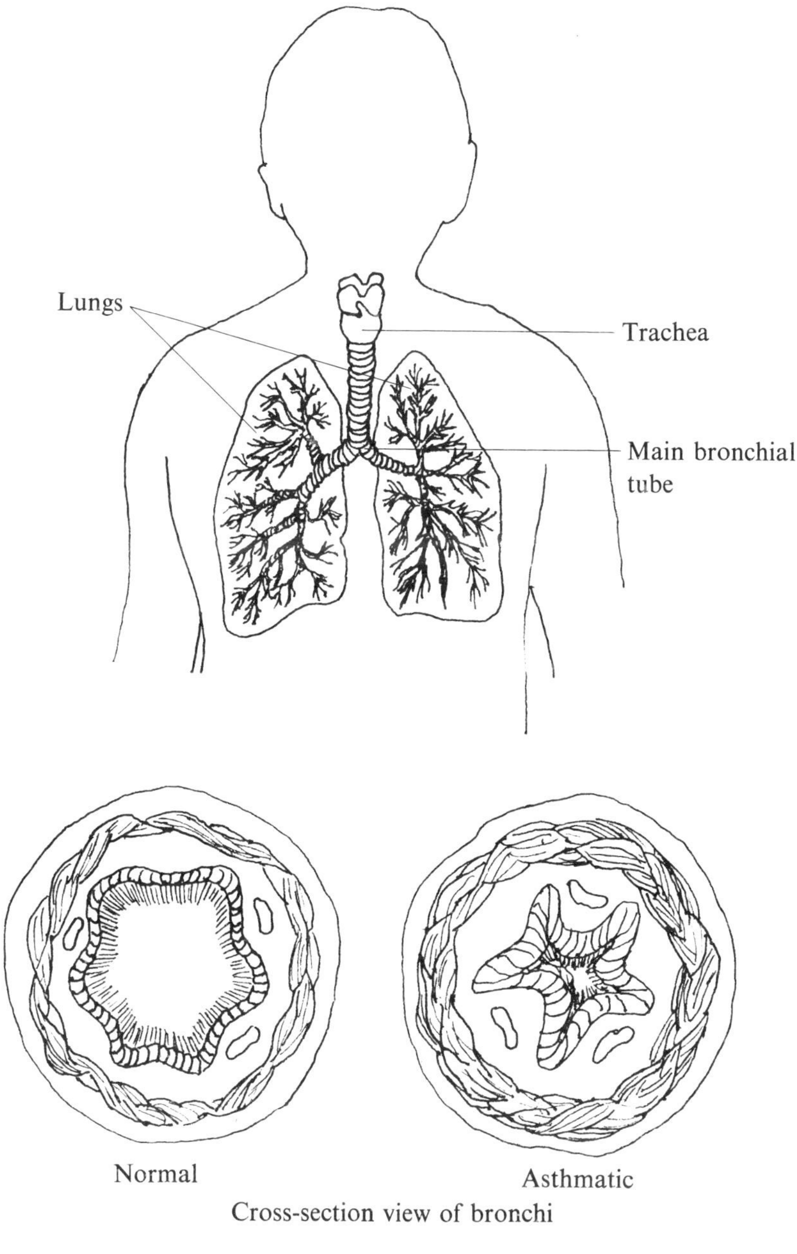

4. *Industrial* or *chemical-induced* asthma, which is stimulated by fumes of epoxy resins and plastics, chemical dusts (platinum), gases (toluene), and other chemicals.

5. *Allergic bronchopulmonary aspergillosis*, which is a special, well-studied type of asthma caused by spores of *Aspergillus fumigatus.*

This classification may seem to make sense on first glance. However when one learns more of the complex underlying mechanisms involved in asthma, one begins to realize that this is a somewhat unjustified over-simplification. With patients of all asthmatic types—immunologic or otherwise—there is hyperreactivity of the bronchial airways to an infinite list of *nonspecific* irritants and broncho-constrictor agents. For example, it is widely recognized that asthma can be precipitated by cold, exercise, and emotional stress. These are nonspecific factors which somehow produce spasms in the already *hyperirritable* bronchi. The real question is: *why* is there this hyperirritability in the first place? Many medical theories have been advanced to explain such hyperreactivity but none are conclusive. As long as these theories adhere to the microscopic and mechanistic way of explanation, they will continue to be too limited.

A more productive orientation would be to consider the common *macroscopic* features of the asthmatic reaction. The most striking macroscopic finding, according to the *Pathologic Basis of Disease*, is obstruction of bronchi and bronchioles by thick, tenacious mucus plugs. These mucus plugs contain whorls of shed *epithelium*, which give rise to the so-called *Curschmann's spirals* and numerous eosinophils. The mucus constituting these plugs is produced in the goblet cells, which line the bronchial tubes. Normally, the cilia move mucus from the bronchial tubes through the trachea. However, in the case of asthma, the goblet cells are over-producing, and mucus accumulates in excess. Initially, as mucus accumulates, there is a gradual narrowing of the bronchial passages. Eventually some of these tubes may be blocked by plugs, and breathing is impeded. In the progression of an attack the person labors to get air into his or her lungs (lung expansion, bronchioles open up) and then cannot exhale (bronchioles more contracted) because of blockage by the plugs. The blocked air passages create the sensation of *dyspnea* or shortness of breath. The wheezing sound characteristic of asthma results from air going through the narrowed passages. During an acute attack, which may last several hours, much of the blood which flows through the walls of the *alveoli* (lung sacs) neither picks up needed oxygen nor gives off carbon dioxide. Obviously, this can have serious adverse effects on our entire body metabolism. The conclusion of an attack is marked by extensive coughing, often bringing up large amounts of mucus. The result of this discharge is considerable relief from the breathing difficulty.

The heavy mucus deposits observed in asthmatic people also serve as a collecting medium for numerous irritants or allergens coming from the environment. The sticky mucus will trap non-specific factors, such as dust, molds, pollen, smoke, and various chemical substances, and these may trigger the asthmatic response. Therefore, the various air pollutants, dust, etc., should not be viewed as primary causes, but as precipitators or triggers of the asthmatic attack. The more solid components of these factors are attracted to and get stuck in the mucus deposits of the bronchial tubes and alveoli. Hence the root of the problem lies in the sticky condition of the bronchial tubes, the alveoli, and blood and capillaries which surround them. Additionally, mucus accumulation in the lungs and bronchi creates other problems which may contribute to the "uncontrollable cycles" of asthmatic attacks. Mucus build-up in the lungs and bronchi may be difficult to discharge if the bronchi are too narrow. Subsequently more and more mucus accumulates, and this causes the alveoli of the lungs to become distended, impairing oxygen absorption of the blood. When the lungs are overburdened in this way, and oxygen absorption is poor, it is not uncommon for moods of depression or sadness to develop. People experiencing such a melancholy state often will seek solace by eating sweet-tasting foods such as ice cream, candy, and soft drinks, all of which enhance mucus accumulation. This cycle may perpetuate itself until the person dies of respiratory exhaustion or heart attack.

We can readily see that the condition of asthma originates in the overconsumption of more yin foods and excessive liquids, since the attack itself entails the discharge of much liquid. Asthma is also frequently associated with many years of overworking kidneys, resulting from the repeated overconsumption of fluids and sugar.

For example, asthmatics may notice that at certain times the attacks come more when they drink more, less when they drink less. They also arise more with wet weather.

There are a number of secondary precipitating factors involved in the asthmatic condition. In addition to wet weather and excessive fluid intake, cold weather will also bring on attacks. These particular factors can encourage both allergic and so-called non-allergic forms of asthma. The non-allergic form is a medical distinction based on the absence of specific antibodies for the offending substance. If the first type (allergic) exists, the asthmatic response is triggered by some environmental factor such as pollen, dust and molds, fish or animal hairs. In the non-allergic type, irritating substances such as fumes, chemical substances and sawdust may also induce the hyperreactive state. So in a more basic or simplistic sense, both types are actually allergic because abnormal sensitivity or intolerance is involved.

Recently there has been much research on the psychosomatic aspects of asthma. Many asthmatics are aware that excessive emotions, such as anger, anxiety, or excitedness, tend to worsen their conditions and sometimes mental tensions will bring on the tightening of bronchial tubes and can actually trigger attacks. Viewing the increasingly stressful life of modern industrial society, it is no wonder that the incidence of asthma has increased so rapidly in the last few decades. The standard American diet, consisting largely of artificial or chemicalized products, as well as refined sugar, flour, and fatty animal food, has lead to serious degeneration of the human nervous sytem. Until recently, people had generally stronger nervous systems and thus were much more adaptable to the stresses of modern industrial life. Due to their strong constitutions these people coped with stress in a beneficial way—that is, their nervous systems were actually strengthened (hence adaptive) by these conditions. But for today's generations, the situation is quite different. Accordingly, some asthmatic treatments incorporate psychotherapy and various psychosomatic techniques directed at controlling emotional upsets which can trigger asthmatic attacks. Such therapies include yoga, dance, biofeedback and visualization. Biofeedback autogenic training and various other forms of "behavior modification" serve primarily to teach the individual to relax and respond appropriately when an attack seems imminent (when wheezing becomes intensified), and therefore can sometimes prevent or delay the onset of an attack. Medical practitioners have begun to integrate behavior modification into the treatment of asthma with some degree of success. However, although the condition is temporarily alleviated by such techniques, asthmatic persons remain dependent on medications which tend to weaken their condition, thus increasing their susceptibility.

Relaxation techniques can be quite useful when integrated with the standard macrobiotic diet, particularly when the individual is becoming independent of prescription drugs. We encourage any form of non-strenuous exercise which keeps the circulatory and respiratory systems running more smoothly; the cleansing processes, especially these of the lymphatic system, are greatly improved by physical exercise.

Cause: Overconsumption of dairy foods, oily and greasy or fatty foods, sugar, sweets and tropical fruits; overconsumption of liquids as well as excessive yin foods. Soft drinks, cold beverages, milk and milk drinks, and fruit juices are often important causes of asthma.

Adjustments to the standard macrobiotic approach: For an initial period of several months, the following suggestions can be incorporated into a general macrobiotic way of eating:

Flour and flour products are best avoided, though again, if desired, a small volume of *seitan*, macrobiotic quality, unyeasted sourdough bread, whole wheat noodles or *fu* may be eaten on occasion. *Vegetables* may all be cooked, with raw salad best avoided; it is especially important to have a good variety of different vegetable dishes, cooked in a variety of ways. The moderate use of *oil* in cooking is appropriate if desired, preferably roasted sesame oil; *nuts and nut or seed butters* are best avoided, though a moderate volume of lightly roasted seeds may be used as a snack or condiment.

A small volume of non-fatty, white-meat *fish* may be eaten once or twice per week if desired. Any type of *beqns* may be used daily or every other day.

Fruits and fruits juices or fruit desserts are best avoided for the initial period; as desired, a small volume of macrobiotic quality, grain- or vegetable-based sweets may be used, though they are best kept to a minimum. The volume of *drinking* may be kept to a comfortable minimum, just enough to satisfy thirst; it is better to avoid cold or chilled beverages.

In addition, the following special dishes can often help to further the progress of relief from asthma: 1) for 1 week, 1/2 cup of the juice from freshly grated lotus root may be heated and drunk daily; or, 2) a small dish of cooked dried lotus or lotus seeds may be eaten daily for one week, and several times per week thereafter; or, 3) lotus root powder cooked with a cup of hot water may be taken daily for five days, and thereafter two or three times per week for about one month.

A mustard plaster or *ginger compress* may be applied to the front and back of the bronchi area several times per week to speed relief. In addition, a person with asthma is advised to avoid cold, wet, damp or humid rooms or climates.

The issue of how soon or how gradually to attempt to withdraw asthma medication is a matter of some sensitivity; even when no more attacks are apparent, they may recur again after several weeks if prompted by a change in environmental factors such as the temperature, emotional stresses, or others. In the event of an attack, a small cup of *kuzu*, sweetened with *amazake* or barley malt syrup can relax the air passages and bring relief. If asthma attacks become too frequent or too severe, it is generally safest to reintroduce the medication and wait an additional period of time before again attempting to withdraw it.

Again, as for hay fever, maintaining a sound digestion and regular elimination is essential to prevent attacks and speed recovery. For recovering from asthma, some form of regular physical exercise is also very helpful in strengthening the circulatory and respiratory system.

3. Food Allergies

Of all the allergies, food allergy stands as the most controversial and interesting for a growing number of doctors, allergists, and immunologists. Its popularity is rapidly spreading, both in terms of diagnoses and as a focus of intellectual interest within medical circles. The actual incidence of food allergy in this country is unknown, mainly because it evades most diagnostic attempts. Food allergy manifests itself across such a grand spectrum of symptoms that it is often misdiagnosed, unrecognized, or (most often) entirely unsuspected. Since everyone has a unique biochemical make-up and therefore has a different range of sensitivity (if susceptible) to the many types of available foods, it is not difficult to see why food allergy can manifest itself in such a diverse array of symptoms. Today this ominous condition is suspected to be the mechanism underlying not only many cases of asthma, rhinitis, skin allergy, and cerebral allergy, but has been linked with a host of other problems affecting all organs and glandular systems. This is not difficult to understand: because our blood carries food particles, metabolites and potential allergens to the skin, respiratory tract and all parts of the body, including the brain.

Food allergy is not a purely modern phenomenon. Hippocrates (460–370 B.C.) reported that cow's milk could cause hives as well as gastric upset. Following him, Galen (A.D. 131–210) described a case of goat's milk allergy. In modern societies allergy to cow's milk is the most common form of allergy among infants and young children. It is also, as one would expect, the most common of food allergies.

The current line of thinking concerning food allergy is that certain foods or food additives which are consumed over a long period of time may sometimes lead to an individual's inability to tolerate these foods. The clinical ecologists have keynoted on the weakening or degeneration of our natural immunity due primarily to the consumption of chemically processed food during pregnancy by the mother, and over generations. This is surely part of the picture, but chemicals or food additives are not the only factors. If they were then how could food allergy have occurred back in ancient Greece in the time of Hippocrates and Galen? Our level of natural immunity or tolerance is determined by a variety of factors associated with diet and lifestyle.

Food-induced allergy can alter our normal immunity in two basic ways. The first is the way most commonly referred to by today's food allergists and immunologists. A person who regularly consumes one type of food over a long period of time has a better chance of developing hypersensitivity to that food than someone who incorporates much variety into their diet. Of course the nutrition received during pregnancy is also important, and predisposes to intolerance in later life. This is especially true if the mother ate large quantities of dairy food, refined carbohydrates, sugar, and chemical-laden food. If the mother feeds her child these same foods as the child develops—the individual will have a tendency to develop food allergy. Many times it will affect the person in early childhood, particularly with foods that are eaten on a regular basis, such as dairy foods, eggs, wheat products, and corn products. Even when the individual adheres to a diet full of variety, if those foods mentioned above are still eaten regularly the tendency to food allergy prevails—although it may not manifest until later in life, or may appear in the form of another allergy, such as asthma or hay fever. Food allergy may also crop up as the covert mechanism behind such digestive disorders as colitis or celiac disease.

This first form of food allergy, which is primarily immunological, affects people either immediately, within several hours, or even days later. The immediate reaction involves the improper digestion of food protein, which then enters the bloodstream in whole form, setting up the sensitization and production of IgE antibodies (similar to hay fever). These antibodies may become attached to mast cells in the digestive and respiratory systems, and also in the skin. Whenever they become attached, various allergic symptoms arise due to the release of histamine. These may include eczema, hives, diarrhea, vomiting, cramps, and nasal irritation and discharge. The delayed food allergy, which is the more common type in children, involves a more complex immune mechanism, but similar symptoms. While both types of reaction may be induced by any kind of food it is usually the richer foods (chocolate, nuts, eggs, fruits, mustard, legumes, tomatoes, sweets, seafood, especially shellfish, and various meats) which trigger the immediate type. The more commonly eaten everyday foods (e.g., dairy foods, wheat and corn products) are more likely to produce the delayed type.

The other form of food allergy, which may be intimately interrelated to the first form, involves a fundamental metabolic deficiency or aberration. Often this occurs because of the lack of a specific enzyme. For example, two components of cow's milk, *caseinogen* and lactose, are often associated with milk allergy. The first, caseinogen, is one of 25 potentially allergenic proteins that have been identified in cow's milk. Caseinogen is difficult to digest or break down properly—and impossible if the necessary enzymes are lacking. The other, lactose, is a simple sugar existing in both cow's milk and human milk that is digested by lactase, an enzyme produced in the intestines. In most traditional societies, lactase is no longer produced after the baby is weaned from its mother's milk—between ages two and four. As a result, ingestion of dairy products produces indigestion, diarrhea, cramps, and various allergic conditions. In our modern society our bodies have adapted to frequent milk drinking by continuing to produce lactase. However, by age 14–16 the lactase enzyme begins to function so poorly that proper metabolism of lactose is minimal. Researchers are now finding a significant degree of lactose intolerance in many cases of milk allergy. In one study lactose intolerance was demonstrated in more than 50 percent of patients with severe gastrointestinal milk allergy.

When today's allergists are confronted with a possible case of food allergy their first instinct is to eliminate cow's milk—no matter what the symptoms are. Unfortunately most food allergists eliminate milk only when someone is shown to be hypersensitive to it by clinical diagnosis; it is then avoided only until the sensitivity is overcome, whereupon it is reintroduced. This is also the conventional approach with other suspected foods. In each case, although the hypersensitivity appears to have been thwarted, it is actually only "masked" and transferred to another part of the body, often to manifest itself in a very different form. Food allergists are aware of this process, but they do not understand the root cause by which to eradicate the inevitable recurrences.

Not all physicians are immune to the suggestion that cow's milk lies at the root of other food sensitivities and of allergies in general. Two doctors, Bahna and Heiner, have recently completed a comprehensive book, *Allergies to Milk*, in which they allude to the possible underlying contribution of cow's milk to general allergic tendencies:

> ". . . Even after apparent disappearance of sensitivity to milk, most patients seem to be "allergy-prone." Later recurrences or the development of other sensitivities are frequent, and new manifestations may be similar to, or different from, the previous symptoms. Whenever symptoms attributable to allergy occur in a subject who previously was known to be allergic to cow's milk but now seems to tolerate it well, the physician must realize that milk may again have a subtle or major role in the patient's new symptoms even though they seem unrelated to the earlier milk-related allergy. Therefore, a trial of reeliminating milk from the diet is always in order because it may significantly contribute to the control of the new allergies." (*Allergies to Milk*, Bahna & Heiner, p. 138, 1980.)

This statement corroborates a number of other findings in which the ingestion of milk led to basic digestive and immunologic disturbances as well as the tendency to develop other food hypersensitivities and new allergies. Some of these studies describe cellular and immunologic abnormalities in the intestinal mucosa which cannot be specifically attributed by clinical diagnosis to cow's milk allergy. These researchers are sometimes compelled to use the term "milk related disorder" rather than simple "milk allergy." Often the terms are used interchangeably, as if there is no disparity.

The confusion commonly experienced by clinical ecologists and other food allergists in interpreting food related problems is due largely to the focus of diagnosis. The usual and most reliable method of diagnosis is the so-called "trial elimination diet." This involves a period of fasting or avoidance of suspected foods (those eaten most regularly), and then gradual reintroduction (testing or "challenge") of each food, one at a time. Most elimination diets initially involve complete abstinence from milk, eggs, chocolate, wheat, corn, legumes, nuts, and cold drinks. This diagnostic test is now held superior over skin tests and blood tests. Sometimes it is used together with a pulse test—if the pulse beat changes dramatically when a food is introduced, that food may be allergenic. Because delayed hypersensitivity may complicate the testing, the individual is advised to keep a detailed record of symptoms prior to and during the trial period. If the testing is carried out carefully and over a period of several weeks the food allergen can usually be identified.

The weakness of this diagnostic approach is its exclusive focus on the "allergenicity" of foods and food additives. The food which is determined as the offending allergen is also established as the "cause." The treatment is accordingly to wipe out or subdue the identified sensitivity food. Unfortunately this is only a superficial treatment, for the offending factor is but a trigger to unleash the cumulative adverse effects of a habitually imbalanced diet. If the food allergen is eliminated, only those symptoms corresponding to that particular allergy disappear. In time, other symptoms will arise which are also likely to be allergic.

The relief of food allergy sometimes takes longer than most other allergies because it may often involve a reordering of one's whole metabolism, as well as rejuvenation of the gastrointestinal tract and immune system. Correct application of the standard macrobiotic diet can usually relieve food allergy within six months. In the case of allergy to whole grains, it may require up to three months until grains can be tolerated comfortably.

It should be noted that the results of food allergy tests are often inaccurate: a test may show, for example, a mild allergic reaction to soybeans or certain grains. Yet, in many cases, when these foods are cooked properly, eaten in balanced combinations and well-chewed, they produce no ill effects. The laboratory testing circumstances, in other words, often do not reflect the reality of balanced eating. An actual adverse reaction to a grain is also often the result of the grain being undercooked, poorly chewed, or eaten in combination with dairy foods, excessive oil, fruit or other sweets, all of which will tend to interfere with the complete digestion of grains if eaten directly together.

The cause: Food allergies are caused primarily by a stagnation of the intestines' functioning, especially caused by long-time consumption of dairy foods. Other foods which contribute to this intestinal stagnation include flour products, particularly yeasted baked flour products, sugar and sweets, oil and oily or greasy foods, tropical fruits and their juices, chemical additives or drugs, and regularly consumed raw salads and other raw foods.

Adjustments to the standard macrobiotic approach: For an initial period of several months, the standard macrobiotic way of eating may be followed, with the general suggestions outlined in the previous chapter in mind. In addition, special care may be taken to have *miso* soup every day, some sea vegetable side dish or dish with a sea vegetable every day, and to chew particularly thoroughly. Some sea vegetable condiment may be used daily, and you may drink 1 cup of *kombu* tea several times a week. Also, one half to one *umeboshi* plum or the equivalent in *shiso* leaves may be used daily as a condiment. Any foods that create a reaction, if normally part of the standard macrobiotic way of eating, may need to be avoided during this initial period until the reaction subsides; these may include wheat, corn, some beans, certain vegetables, or others. After about three months, the allergic person may sample a small portion of the triggering food to see if the reaction has disappeared. The relief of food allergies may take somewhat longer than for most other allergies, as the individual's entire metabolism may need to reorder itself. Correct application of this way of eating can usually relieve any food allergies within four to six months. In the case of allergies to whole grains, it may require several months until the grain or grains can be tolerated. During this time, the other grains can be relied upon.

4. Skin Allergies: Hives, Angioedema and Eczema

Skin allergy is a general term referring collectively to those allergies which manifest in an altered skin condition. In the field of allergy, skin allergy poses a great challenge, because it is believed to be caused by virtually anything. Both hives and eczema have been linked with food allergy (particularly to eggs, shellfish, nuts, or fruits), all varieties of medication, chemicals, pollens, insect stings, sunlight, cold temepratures, infections, parasites, exercise, and certain illnesses of adjustment. There has been a great deal of inaccuracy in the treatment of skin allergy, since the trigger may come from the inside as well as from outside, and skin tests are rarely helpful. In most cases doctors admit that the cause may never be found.

Skin disease is not merely a problem with the skin itself—all types of skin disease are also different manifestations of some internal imbalance. The most common causes of skin disorders are animal foods—e.g., meat, eggs, dairy, and fish—followed by sugar, fruit juice, oil, and other expansive foods. When approaching skin disease, we should ideally not try to suppress this discharge, but allow it to come out while at the same time eliminating the cause of the problem.

Like all skin disease, hives and eczema serve the invaluable function of discharging excess (toxins, fluids, etc.), which has accumulated internally in and around various organs, as well as throughout the digestive and lymphatic systems. The discharge of toxins permits the internal organs and tissues to continue functioning smoothly. Since the intestines are the first to be affected, it is especially important to work initially at strengthening their functions. Weak intestines will lead to poor absorption of nutrients, and elimination will be forced through the skin. Other internal structures that are adversely affected during the course of skin allergy are the kidneys, liver and thyroid gland. The kidneys are weakened by milk and milk products, sugar, fruits, chemicals and very strong drugs (e.g., antibiotics and various pharmaceuticals). The liver is weakened by overconsumption of animal foods, sugar, and by the more gradual, long-term effects of ingesting chemicals or food additives. The diminished functioning of both organs results in an over-acidic and polluted blood condition, accompanied by mucus and fat deposits throughout the lymphatic system. These mucus deposits not only hinder the filtering functions of the lymphatic network, but also attract the IgE antibodies which participate in allergic reactions. When the IgE collect in these areas of excess, the ensuing discharge allows for the release of extra fluids, and hence the temporary relief of an overly expanded, watery condition. The third structure, the thyroid gland, is usually not considered in allergic reactions. However, this endocrine gland controls the functions of the three layers of skin. When these regulatory functions are impaired, the skin's inner layers, the *serous* and *mucous* membranes, are forced to eliminate excess fluids and toxins when provoked by even the mildest allergic reaction. The thyroid's deterioration often parallels that of the kidneys and liver, and underlies many cases of abnormal elimination through the skin. Until the kidneys, liver, lungs and intestines have regained their collective capacity for eliminating toxins, the thyroid will become overworked and weakened—until eventually even the skin begins to fail as the last resort for discharging excess. If this stage is reached more severe degeneration such as skin cancer may become evident.

Hives, also known as *urticaria*, is characterized by itchy skin with bumps or "wheals" of varying size. These wheals are raised and pale, and are often surrounded by an area of redness and warmth. Such localized swelling or edema is due to clogged lymphatic channels and, subsequently, fluid accumulation. Hives involves both an allergic reaction and an over-expanded and weakened lymphatic system. The reaction entails the release of histamine from the numerous mast cells throughout our skin. Histamine has a dual effect: (1) dilation of small blood vessels under the skin, thereby increasing permeability to allow the leaking out or excretion of a clear serum; and (2) irritation of nerve endings to bring on itchy, reddened skin. The first effect constitutes a process of discharge whereas the second is a message which tells us that we have been overindulging in sugar, sweets, fruits, dairy foods, raw foods, and liquids.

In hives, the overexpanded and weakened condition of organs, glands, tissues, and the peripheral nervous system can be irritated by a variety of physical factors. Sunlight, which has a yangizing effect, will often stimulated the elimination of excess fluids, sugars, and other yin elements through the skin. In opposite manner, cold temepratures, make the blood vessels contract, forcing the discharge by pressure. Physical exercise serves a similar, contracting function, so mild forms (e.g., walking, yoga, swimming, and *t'ai chi chuan*) will further encourage the discharge and accelerate recovery.

In addition, hives may be precipitated by emotional upsets such as are characteristic with people who have consumed many fruits, liquids, food additives, milk products, and sweet or sugary foods. Sugar tends to make people fluctuate between hyperactivity and depression or other emotional instability. The combination of milk and sugar instigates an overall weakening of the autonomic nervous functions, in addition to those of the kidneys, spleen, thyroid, and pancreas. An over-acidic blood condition will potentiate the inflammation or swelling of peripheral nerve cells, and emotional imbalances often accompany this process. In addition, the lack of adequate amounts of B-vitamins, caused by overconsumption of white sugar or other refined carbohydrates, will make the central nervous system malfunction, paving the way for over-excited, excessively sensitive, and temperamental behavior. Also, allergic spasm or dilation of important arteries in the head that supply the brain is often caused by various processed foods, chemicals, or food additives, leading to moodiness and other abnormal emotional behavior. By eating primarily whole grains, beans, vegetable soups, and land and sea vegetables the nervous system is restored to a more harmonious state. Social or family support and a harmonious environment will greatly facilitate this strengthening process.

Angioedema, like hives, involves eruption, but with more diffuse swelling of loose subcutaneous (below the skin surface) tissue. This more generalized allergic reactions often associated with swelling of the lips, tongue, eyelids, throat, mucous membranes, and sex organs. The condition is caused more by prolonged consumption of extremely expansive foods such as sugar, alcohol, tropical fruits, and fruit juices in addition to chemically processed foods and food additives. Angioedema is more commonly preceded or instigated by food allergy. The gastrointestinal tract is functioning very poorly, and nausea, vomiting, colic, and intestinal obstruction are common. The upper respiratory tract is secondarily affected, sometimes leading to fatal blockage of the upper airways in a manner similar to asthma.

Hives usually precedes angioedema, which is a more serious form of anaphylaxis. With this disorder the body is forced to spread out the process of discharge since more organs and tissues are being adversely affected. The kidneys, bladder, lungs, and large intestine are functioning so poorly that the entire skin surface must be utilized to eliminate excess. Cold weather and emotional stress will further aggravate the condition. In this case, very simple and moderate eating is essential.

The third type of atopic skin problem is *eczema*. This condition is characterized by itchy, red, and dry skin, and may be chronic or acute. Eczema may occur either as an allergy or as a general hyperreaction to irritating or toxic substances. The nonallergic type usually involves direct skin contact with irritants such as detergents, insecticides, herbicides, and industrial chemicals. The allergy type involves an aberration or deficiency in some specific immune response, either internally (affecting various organs and tissues) or externally (upon skin contact with an allergen). Because the internal triggers are usually not revealed by conventional diagnosis, the patient seeks to alleviate the condition with moisturizing and softening creams and cortisone ointments applied directly over the skin.

The eczematic person has the same general dietary history which tends to produce other skin disorders. This primarily includes dairy foods, sugar and sweet-tasting foods, but also the excessive intake of baked flour products, fruits, oily or greasy foods, and chemically processed foods. The dry condition is caused by accumulations of fat and mucus directly under the skin and in the lymphatic and digestive systems as a result of general overeating, and prolonged consumption of oily or fatty foods (e.g., pizza, french fries, and hamburger) and baked foods. The itchy skin characteristically reflects the declining quality of the peripheral nervous system.

Eczema is a common disease of infancy often observed in the first few weeks of life, reflecting greatly imbalanced eating habits throughout the mother's pregnancy. Most cases of eczema are apparent by the age of two years. During this time the development of the immune and digestive systems are in constant flux, depending on the relative balance of expansive and contractive foods in the mother's and post-breastfed baby's diet. Harmonious eating during this time is fundamental to the prevention of eczema. In subsequent years, eczema will also involve impaired functioning of the respiratory system, and individuals frequently develop respiratory allergies such as hay fever and asthma.

Cause: In general, skin allergies are caused by the long-term overconsumption of dairy foods, oily and greasy foods, sugar, sweets, refined flour and other refined grain products, tropical foods and beverages, spices, drugs and chemical additives; in addition, certain animal foods often play an important role, including eggs, poultry, red-meat or blue-skinned fish.

Adjustments to the standard macrobiotic approach: The daily *way of cooking* may be fully varied, including both more well-cooked and more lightly cooked dishes; all salt taste and salt seasoning may be mild. A dish of *nishime* style vegetables should be used every other day.

Flour and baked flour products are best avoided; whole wheat noodles, an occasional slice of macrobiotic quality bread, *fu* and *seitan* may occasionally be used if desired, though it is best to avoid buckwheat flour, such as buckwheat or *soda* noodles. Raw salads are also best avoided; a boiled salad can be used if there is a craving for salad.

Beans, preferably only *azuki*, lentil and chickpea, may be used often but in small, amounts only. The use of *oil*, nuts, nut and seed butters is best minimized; high quality, roasted sesame oil may be used if desired once or twice per week in cooking; and if desired, a small volume of white-meat, non-fatty *fish* may be eaten once or twice per week, cooked together with leafy green vegetables. *Pumpkin and sesame seeds* may be used regularly, but sunflower seeds are better avoided.

Fruit and fruit desserts and juices are best avoided entirely, though a small volume of cooked fruit may be tolerated very occasionally if desired. If desired, also, macrobiotic grain and vegetable desserts may be used to satisfy sweet cravings. A cup of boiled *azuki* juice with a pinch of sea salt added may be taken daily for 3–7 weeks.

In addition to diet, an important factor in relieving skin allergies is to try and minimize direct contact with artificial clothing and environments. Synthetic or woolen clothing can irritate the skin and easily trigger an allergic reaction. Whenever possible, garments worn directly next to the skin can be of cotton; and all synthetic or irritating cosmetics may be kept to a minimum.

To help alleviate the symptoms of any skin eruption, a simple plaster made of raw, fine-chopped greens, rice bran or green *nori* flakes, and enough white flour to hold the mixture together as a paste, may be spread out over a cheesecloth or cotton backing and applied to the affected area.

5. Chemical Allergy

In this world of expanding petrochemical industrialization and technological advancements to improve "standards of living," the release of large amounts of harmful chemicals into our environment is becoming an increasing health hazard. Besides the pollutants circulating in much of our air and water, thousands of chemical additives have entered the commercial food market, thereby allowing long distance food transportation and longer shelf-life. Additives have also been produced to give new sensorial dimensions to food such as new tastes, textures, colors and smells. With the Space Age giving birth to more and more convenience foods and synthetic foods, it would seem that in a very short time, perhaps by A.D. 2000, all of what we now call "natural foods" will be regarded by the majority as extreme luxuries, or at best as remnants of an old-fashioned age. Even for people who assert themselves as following a certain "natural diet," there's a good chance that some of their produce contains significant traces of fertilizer, herbicide, or pesticide—unless the items are grown organically.

Our chemical environment is of both a strengthening and a potentially harmful nature, depending on the extent of our natural immunity. Some individuals remain immune to serious illness even though they consume large amounts of extreme foods and are exposed to toxic chemicals in their environment. Why is this so? Usually, the individuals' inherited constitutions are very strong and well-built, rich in various minerals. Their mothers and forebears ate plenty of grains and hearty vegetables and passed along sound digestive, circulatory, and nervous systems that can withstand heavy abuse. Other people who do not necessarily have strong constitutions but who appear immune to illness frequently have unusually strong day-to-day energy and vitality from activities and exercises, which they have cultivated over many years of balanced living. These people too can absorb and neutralize almost any extreme factor up to a certain point.

For example, in Nagasaki following the atomic bombing in August 1945, a group of surviving macrobiotic doctors and patients avoided radiation sickness by eating brown rice, sea salt, *miso* soup, sea vegetables, and other very yang traditional foods. Meanwhile, many other survivors in Nagasaki eating the modern Japanese diet of white rice, heavy animal food, and sugar died of radiation sickness within a few days or of leukemia in subsequent years.

Modern industrial societies are experiencing an unprecedented need for a way of life and eating practices which create strong natural immunity. The constant exposure to harmful pollution in urban, suburban and rural districts also poses a serious menace to the biological and psychological well-being of the city's inhabitants. As a consequence of the growing constitutional weaknesses of most young people, due to improper nourishment during embryonic development, the spread of diseases once ascribed to "old-age" are now afflicting many of the younger generations. Some of these, once problems of old-age, include cancer, arthritis, cataracts, atherosclerosis, and impotence or sterility. This trend is a clear indication of the degeneration and vulnerability of modern society as a whole.

By conservative estimates, according to Samuel Epstein, M.D., in *The Politics of Cancer*, the average American eats nine pounds of chemical additives a year including preservatives, flavoring agents, stabilizers, and artificial colors. Therefore over several decades of such dietary practice the individual will have received several hundred pounds of food additives. Chemical agriculture and fast food industries are generating a whirlpool of artificial chemical elements which is making the modern diet increasingly inappropriate for human consumption.

With about three thousand synthetic and natural chemicals now being used for preserving, coloring, flavoring and stabilizing prepared foods, many allergy-prone individuals are increasingly apt to develop chemical allergy. The chemicals may trigger an allergic reaction in very complex ways; for example, they can either react individually, or synergistically with other chemicals. Because of the gigantic range of possible mechanisms and potential risks accompanying the ingestion of chemically adulterated foods, chemical technologists and food allergy specialists are compelled to speculate a great deal about the harmfulness of these food products, although, they may happily relate the benefits of the additives in terms of improved flavor, shelf-life, etc. In many cases, if additives are held suspect as the "cause," the hypersensitive person will be placed on an additive-free diet—that is, on any type of food which is devoid of synthetic chemicals. Such people, often lacking understanding of their total nutritional needs, will search out additive-free dairy products, eggs, meats, concentrated sweeteners, vegetables and fruits. The problem here is that people will continue to take the foods which support their underlying susceptibility to other allergic reactions: milk, milk-products, and sugary foods.

The more severe cases of chemical allergy reflect deeply disturbed or imbalanced metabolic and immunologic functions. Such people may have violent reactions to infinitesimally small amounts of chemical gases and dusts or other allergens. Only a few molecules, or a one part-per-billion dilution of some chemical, may be all that is needed to stimulate the allergic reaction. These are the cases by which allergists are continually frustrated. Usually the only effective medical approach is to provide a sterile, "allergen-free" environment, and to limit food consumption to one or two foods per day on a "rotation diet." The patient is often so sensitive that not even allergy drugs can be used. Many such people must wear oxygen masks whenever they step out of their house, and their entire environment, whether natural or unnatural, becomes an omnipresent opponent to be feared and despised.

In view of the extremely delicate, sensitive nature of this type of condition, it is especially advisable for such a hypersensitive individual to seek the counsel of an experienced macrobiotic advisor when beginning the macrobiotic approach. If the person with intense chemical allergies maintains a very well ordered, balanced macrobiotic diet and daily way of living, particularly with qualified guidance, recovery will come eventually. No allergic condition is permanent unless the affected individual does not believe that he can change himself. We create our state of illness and discomfort ourselves, and we can just as well create our highest health and happiness.

There is to date no other approach which can completely relieve the devastating condition of someone with extreme chemical allergies. For the most renowned specialists this immunologic disorder remains as one of the most baffling mysteries.

6. Cerebral Allergy

Some types of allergies appear to bring about dramatic behavior and mood changes. Although there is no evidence that allergic reactions per se occur in the brain tissue, the term *cerebral allergies* is used because the symptoms (somehow) affect the brain and nervous system. People who are said to have cerebral allergy will evidence depression, neurosis, psychosis, or schizophrenia. The primary symptoms in most cases are anxiety and depression, but dizziness, blurred vision, catatonia, paranoid delusions, and hallucinations also occur. Often, when these people are subjected to a series of highly sophisticated diagnostic tests, a specific food allergy is discovered. In such cases, if the offending food(s) is eliminated, the mental disturbances abate. However, if, as in many cases, the food or chemical allergen remains unidentified, the individual is unfortunately compelled to spend the rest of his life labeled as "mentally ill." Many allergists suspect that a great many psychosis cases in America are food-related cerebral allergies. Work with juvenile delinquent homes has indicated that so-called cerebral food allergy may be underlying a considerable amount of hyperactivity and learning disorders among children.

How can food or food additives induce such extreme, immediate, and uncontrollable emotional reactions in certain individuals? Again, we should first realize that the suspected allergen is not the root cause. If this were true we should all very soon have to label ourselves mentally ill or manic depressive. The offending food or chemical element is only a trigger for cerebral allergy. The real issue, again, is the abnormal physiologic quality of the immune, nervous, and digestive systems, which collectively creates the underlying predisposition to cerebral food allergy.

When cerebral allergy occurs, the only distinct observation of physical change is spasm and/or expansion of the blood vessels, particularly in the forebrain, or frontal area of the head. This tendency toward expansion or dilation reflects an extremely yin condition of the central nervous system, as well as of the body as a whole. In many cases this overly-expanded condition is due to a dietary history of refined carbohydrate foods, chemical additives, drugs, nightshade vegetables, soft drinks, and tropical fruits and fruit juices. Dairy foods taken since early childhood, along with plenty of other animal foods, will provide the foundation for this abnormal condition.

The brain and intestines share a very special complementary and antagonistic relationship. The brain receives vibrational food in the form of waves or radiation, while the intestines receive physical food from the vegetable, animal and mineral kingdoms. If we overeat, our intestines become expanded and do not absorb food very well. Simultaneously our thinking becomes dull or sluggish, as the intestines draw blood (and oxygen) away from the brain. When digestion goes smoothly and the quality of food is properly balanced, our mind is alert, clear and positive. A fine network of meridians and nerves connects the brain to the intestines, picking up very fine or subtle signals between the two organs. Accordingly, when the intestines constrict in the case of an allergic reaction to food, the brain elicits the complementary-opposite response of expansion or *vasodilation*. Extremely expansive foods such as white sugar, spices, alcohol, vitamin C, and drugs, will cause the parasympathetic nervous system to respond erratically wherever allergic reactions occur. The autonomic nervous system and digestive system are completely interdependent in their respective functions and states of health. By regulating our eating habits we can bring these systems back into their natural, harmonious relationship.

7. Rh Incompatibility

The blood of many people contains a substance known as the *Rh factor*. The name "Rh" came from the Rhesus monkey, which was used in the initial experiments connected with this problem. Rh is one of many blood group antigens found on the surface of red blood cells which appears to take part in a peculiar form of allergic reaction. The Rh factor, called *Rh positive*, (in about 85 percent of the population) acts as an *agglutinogen*, which means that it causes a clumping together of red blood cells If the Rh factor is missing the blood is described as *Rh negative*. When Rh positive blood is transfused into someone with Rh negative, the body of the recipient produces an anti-Rh agglutinogen (antibody which attacks the Rh positive cells), usually within two weeks after the transfusion. Serious difficulties may arise if this person is given a second transfusion. The presence of this anti-agglutinogen results in a *hemolytic reaction*, or the destruction of red blood cells, which can be fatal.

The more common problem of today involves Rh incompatibility between the fetus and mother during pregnancy. This results from fertilization of an Rh negative woman's egg by an Rh positive man's sperm. If the embryo inherits the man's Rh factor, its blood will become Rh positive. When this happens, the Rh negative woman may produce the anti-Rh factor as a defense mechanism, since fetal Rh factors are likely to enter the mother's bloodstream. In a subsequent pregnancy, the baby may experience a hemolytic reaction in which its red blood cells are destroyed. Anemia, jaundice, heart failure or other fatal symptoms may result.

Since the Rh factor produces a gathering-in process (agglutination), Rh positive blood is under the influence of centripetal or yang energy, while Rh negative is governed more by centrifugal or yin energy. When Rh positive blood is transfused into Rh negative, the anti-Rh factor arises. This means that the more yin blood quality can tolerate only a small amount of the yang blood quality. In this case, however, with a second transfusion, the blood of the recipient becomes very yang, triggering the hemolytic reaction. This happens because the red blood cells cannot tolerate this second influx of yang since like charges repel each other. In order to balance this, the red blood cells suddenly expand and decompose (a yin process).

The Rh factor of the blood can be changed more easily through proper eating than can the blood type (types O, A, B and AB). This is because blood type reflects a person's constitution, whereas the Rh factor represents the condition. Through dietary adjustment, Rh positive blood can become Rh negative and vice versa. However, if a mother wishes to make her blood Rh positive or more neutral, it is advisable to practice the macrobiotic way of eating for at least four or five years before deciding on having a second child with an Rh positive father (who should also eat macrobiotically). The medical alternative is to inject *RhoGAM*, a conglomeration of special Rh antibodies which suppresses the Rh negative mother's violent immune response to the foreign Rh positive red blood cells that may be produced by the fetus. So far there appear to be no adverse side-effects accompanying the use of RhoGAM.

For mothers who have only recently been introduced to the macrobiotic way of eating, it may be more auspicious to have RhoGAM injected. It should be realized, however, that while this medical approach appears to cause no immediate harm, by its very usage we are ignoring the fundamental issue of Rh positive and Rh negative differentiation. Recently the number of people with Rh positive blood has been increasing. Differentiation of each Rh group is directly influenced by present eating patterns. In other words, the modern diet is extreme on both sides (e.g., meat and sugar), producing a more extreme electromagnetic charge in each Rh group. Close to 50 percent of the average daily diet in America is comprised of animal foods, including dairy. This necessitates eating large quantities of refined carbohydrates to make balance. Usually large amounts of simple sugar—either in the form of refined cane sugar, corn syrup, maple sugar, refined flour and fruits—are used to achieve this. However, if we eat a more balanced or neutral diet our blood reflects this balance and the Rh factor will be neither strongly positive nor negative. If you receive a transfusion under these circumstances, an extreme reaction between plus and minus factors should not arise. In this case the difference between the blood of a mother and her baby will not be great enough to produce an extreme reaction. Persons not eating properly, or only partially following the macrobiotic diet, should be very careful about this problem.

8. Autoimmune Disease

Hypersensitivity to the outside world or to environmental factors (food, drugs, mold, etc.) is the most common conception of allergy. However, hypersensitivity can also be directed toward the internal environment as well—to the body's own cells and tissues. In this more extreme form of allergy, the body manufactures an antibody that is hyperreactive or intolerant toward its own tissues and/or circulating cells, including the basic protein of *myelin* (the nerve fiber insulator), antigens of the thyroid gland, the testicles, stomach gastric cells, platelets, and others. *Autoimmune* diseases differ from other forms of allergy in that their mechanism involves abnormal T-cells as well as abnormal B-cells. In the allergies discussed so far, the quality of the B-cell is the determining factor for abnormally high sensitivity. But in autoimmune disease the T-cell plays an equally fundamental role. B-cells need the help (regulation) of T-cells to differentiate into antibody-secreting cells. Therefore, autoimmune diseases in which the activation of B-cells is somehow altered are linked with derangements in the quality of T-cells also.

Autoimmunity is a general term which describes the body's immunologic and complex way of maintaining a state of equilibrium for the immune system. Infections, injuries, or other temporary disturbances are accompanied by both immune (antibodies) and autoimmune (autoantibodies) responses, both of which serve to keep the body in balance. Mammals must have sufficient autoimmunity to carry on their highly sophisticated protective processes. Simply speaking, autoimmunity is the body's proper discriminating response toward "self" and "non-self." When the immune (autoimmune) system fails to recognize self, it attacks a variety of the body's constitutents and all other normal immune functions are disrupted.

Autoimmune diseases, which may include multiple sclerosis, pancreatitis, pernicious anemia, hepatitis, rheumatoid arthritis, various kidney disorders, and other illnesses, are becoming much more common in today's affluent societies. Often the abnormal immune response is triggered by a viral or bacterial infection. Again, as in other forms of allergy, the antibodies are of an "abnormal" quality, although they may appear to be physically similar to other, normal antibodies. *Thrombocytopenia* is an autoimmune disease characterized by internal hemorrhage, in which blood platelets are either inadequately produced or increasingly destroyed by the abnormal antibodies (deranged autoantibodies). Such illnesses are usually handled with the use of powerful drugs (such as cortisone), or, as in the case of thrombocytopenia, by removal of the spleen and various lymph nodes. In many cases the drugs do not sufficiently interfere with abnormal antibody production or action, so surgery and alternative therapies (blood transfusion, heavy doses of vitamin C, etc.), are necessitated. Whatever the therapy, the end result is inevitably a serious weakening of one's natural immunity and therefore a great likelihood of developing another serious illness in later life.

Unless these diseases are understood in terms of their fundamental cause, they will continue to proliferate and jeopardize the lives of millions of people. In macrobiotic terms, autoimmune diseases result from either one of two ways of extreme eating: (1) overconsumption of excessively expansive (yin) foods; and (2) overconsumption of both strong yin and strong yang foods. Arthritis, for example, which may sometimes involve a faulty autoimmune mechanism, is most often caused by excessive intake of various yin foods such as fruits, fruit juice, especially tropical and semi-tropical varieties, spices, stimulants and aromatic herbs and beverages, soft drinks, sugar, honey, chocolate, and vinegars, as well as excessive intake of tomato, eggplant, and other vegetables of tropical origin. The other form of arthritis is due to excessive consumption of primarily yang foods, including meat, poultry, eggs, hard cheeses, and other animal foods, and large amounts of salt and other minerals. Both forms involve, as a foundation, excessive or long-term consumption of dairy foods and refined sugars. Ice cream and highly-processed dairy foods are basic causes to all forms of autoimmune disease. Drugs, megavitamin therapies, alcohol, ionizing radiation, estrogen and other very expansive factors will induce or potentiate autoimmune diseases. Clinical manifestations are often characterized by the presence of purplish or brownish red skin discolorations (*purpura*), which are eliminations of past excess of simple sugars and other yin dietary factors.

For all forms of serious allergy, such as autoimmune disease, one should initially seek the guidance of a qualified macrobiotic counselor.

9. Christmas Trees

The current medical view of allergies is that anybody can react abnormally to anything—but all for obscure reasons. In Chapter 2 of their recent book, *The Best Guide to Allergies*, three medical doctors and a medical researcher include a section on Christmas trees. The authors point out that many people are sensitive to pollens from trees that can be either standing or cut down (such as Christmas trees). According to these scientists:

> "Recent studies have indicated that a specific allergenic chemical, *terpene*, is released by the tree itself. This substance directly causes allergy symptoms of nasal congestion and discharge and wheezing in a sensitized individual." (*The Best Guide to Allergies*, p. 22)

Should we be relieved and proud of the fact that the "allergenic" substance has been identified? The only ones who will benefit from such information are the huge pharmaceutical industries, who will isolate the terpene compound in order to develop a drug which specifically suppresses the abnormal immune response. Their advertisement would appropriately include a Christmas scene, with gifts under a Christmas tree, and the caption: "The perfect gift for every Christmas." But what if a drug were not discovered? Or if the family decided that trips to the allergy specialist were too expensive? Then, instead of real trees, the family would buy an artificial one, and the problem would be "solved." Of course, the allergic person remains allergic, in spite of the millions spent nationwide each year to promote nasal sprays, antihistamines, bronchodilators, allergy shots, and the many other symptomatic approaches—even artificial Christmas trees! If the same individual finds himself allergic to bee pollen the following spring, will he not then seek to eliminate the bees? The allergic person should understand that it is he—not nature—who is out of balance.

Conclusion—The Restoration of Biological Society

Today, as our civilization reaches an unprecedented level of material wealth and luxurious living, hundreds of millions of people, rich and poor, young and old, educated and uneducated, continue to suffer from cancer, allergies, arthritis, diabetes, and many other serious disorders. Each year new scientifically engineered therapies hold the promise of relief, only to be met with the discovery of undesirable side-effects, long-term inefficiency, or some other defect. For instance, in an increasing number of cases, allergy results as a hypersensitivity to some element of the medication itself! Allergy is fast becoming one of the most widespread and confounding modern diseases for healthcare practitioners around the globe.

The prevailing view is that anything can cause allergy. And, since allergy can manifest in myriad ways—from the usual itchy, runny nose and eyes to canker sores to migraine headaches to epileptic fits—the prevailing view has become "Anything can cause anything." A single allergen, whatever its form, can cause 15 or more different reactions in as many people. The allergy specialist is thus compelled to try a range of complicated sensitivity challenge tests each time someone comes with an obscure allergy problem.

The study of allergic phenomena in all areas of healthcare today is moving along two divergent paths. On one hand there are those strictly concerned with the immunological mechanism of the allergic reaction and its particular corresponding effects. For example, hay fever has led such specialists to a more complex analysis of the nose, and of the related mechanisms and, classifications of nasal disease. They acknowledge the effects created within the nose as elicited by allergic (stimuli) brought through the blood and nervous system. If through the blood circulation, the "cause" of the reaction is food allergens transferred from the intestines. If through the nervous system, the cause may be attributed to an obscure "derangement" of the parasympathetic nerve supply; oftentimes a psychological cause is suspected, or perhaps an "innate" imbalance in brain chemistry. In this latter case, psychotherapy sessions are often pursued and hypnosis or autogenic training are common practices.

On the other side, there are those healers devoted to locating the underlying biological cause of allergy. This latter group regards the disorder not as an isolated chemical reaction on the cellular level, but as the biological consequence of an upset or imbalanced internal environment. Now the issue becomes a matter of varying perspectives, and the allergic person is faced with a confusing maze of options. First visiting the local nutritionist, he is told that his allergies are due to a lack of vitamin C and various other vitamins, so high dosages are prescribed as a cure. When that approach proves insufficient, he visits the chiropractor who tells him that the altered resistance is due to interference in the nervous system, caused by a bone out of its proper position. Some years after he seeks a homeopath, who optimistically offers several remedies for his condition. Then comes the herbalist, then the acupuncturist, and then, finally back to another reputable nutritionist to relieve him of the persistent menace. During this entire time of searching, he may have experienced many temporary successes—intermittent periods of joyful freedom—only to have the allergy stubbornly resurface, sometimes in a completely different form. In spite of the many approaches that have been tried, not one has been able to completely clear the body of allergic vulnerability. The root cause has been nothing less than a medical enigma for conventional and alternative doctors alike.

Since allergies stem from an environmental cause as well as constitutional tendencies, everyone is, to some degree, potentially allergic. If everyone has the capacity to be allergic, what makes some people allergic but others not? Why do boys tend to develop atopic asthma more than girls? Why is it that in temperate zones this kind of asthma occurs more frequently in children born in late autumn or early winter than in other seasons? Why is there a greater likelihood of becoming allergic if complications arose during the birthing process? Why does hernia often accompany respiratory allergies? Why do bananas, papayas, honeydew melon and other sweet tropical fruits appear to "potentiate" allergic reactivity in many cases? And finally, why is the blame continually placed on dust and bees, dogs and cats, forest and field, clouds and rain, slow birth and ripe bananas?

For the reason that one can become allergic to virtually anything in the environment, allergy may be considered a form of biological insanity. Without a comprehensive understanding of the universal order of life, none of the above puzzles can be completely solved, and relentless expansion of allergic disorders will continue to foil even the most advanced medical approaches. For the recovery of millions of people from this present day current of biological schizophrenia, we need a total approach, initiated through our own deep self-reflection upon our way of life, and upon the orientation of our civilization as a whole. The macrobiotic way of life, including its dietary practice, is the most certain way to approach allergy.

6. Personal Experiences

Hay Fever: Mark Mead, Portland, Oregon

My family and I have lived on our New Hampshire farm for eight years. During this time we have had cows, horses, sheep, goats, chickens, dogs, and cats. In the first few years my job was to milk the cows, and to manage the dairy business in general, including maintenance and milk sales. Whenever there was surplus, my five brothers and sisters and I could easily drink it up. I recall sitting down with my brothers and sharing a gallon of the fresh Jersey milk between the three of us—the farmwork gave us big appetites. Besides, who could resist such sweet, high quality milk?

After a few years, I began to notice a pattern of intense reactions whenever I was working in the fields, and, especially when working around the cows. Eventually, I realized that I had severe hay fever, and also that I had a strange sensitivity to the cows themselves, or to cow hair dust or dander. Often within a few minutes of sitting down to do the milking I was plagued with relentless sneezing, and incessant clogging and irritation of the sinuses. I would emerge from the barn red-faced, with eyes and nose dripping. In spite of all this suffering, I refused to tell anyone else about my allergies.

When my family decided to try macrobiotics about four years ago, in the early spring of 1981, I had no intention of curing my allergies. However, within three months all hay fever symptoms had disappeared, my tolerance to cows grew steadily. Eventually we sold all our animals, as our farming and nutritional interests shifted to vegetable gardening and rice growing. I can now be working out in a hay field or in a musty, dusty barn and never have a reaction. The food is clearly centering and energizing. Once your body gets a real taste of it, it never forgets the lightness, altertness and flexibility characteristic of sound health.

Now that the allergic condition has passed, I notice how much life I had been missing out on—on being able to play, completely and endlessly in whatever I do. Also, I notice that I'm meeting allergic people everyday, so I can see there is a great need for a genuine, effective solution to this problem. In order to change, a person must be willing to observe life from a larger perspective, to see him- or herself as an integral but infinitesimal part of nature's myriad cycles. The real purpose of macrobiotics, it seems to me, is not curing sickness, but learning how to live in constant peace and happiness.

Allergies: Mari Kennedy-Metz, Portland, Oregon

For most of my life I was plagued with sinus problems and allergies. In fifth grade I was so sick and exhausted all the time that in early winter I was hospitalized for 5 days in order to undergo a battery of tests, including those for anemia and leukemia. Nothing could be found, however, and my maladies were eventually labeled "virus." Treatment consisted of vitamin B shots, a tonic to encourage my meager appetite, and occasional antibiotic pills. It seemed that I was always out of school (40 to 60 days a year) and at the doctor's office.

My pediatrician finally decided that my cat was at the root of the problem and recommended getting rid of her. I'd gotten her shortly after my Dad died and since I had no friends I could not accept losing her, too. However, she was banished to the basement and never allowed in the house after that. My diet up to that time had consisted largely of fudge bars, ice cream, pop, fast foods, TV dinners, cakes, potato chips, white flour, and frequent dinners out.

The discouraging part was that none of the treatment I received really helped me. I had sinus pressure and headaches constantly, a runny nose, frequent colds, severe intestinal cramping, alternating constipation and diarrhea, frequent nausea and vomiting. I was so exhausted that I literally had to force myself to get up and go to bed—I had *no* energy. Iowa's winters were very hard for me, also. I had two spots in the house where I would spend most of my time sitting: in front of the register in the bathroom, or in front of the register in the living room. I was always cold, even though our house was heated to 80 degrees F. or better much of the time. I was so embarrassed at having to go everywhere with a kleenex in my hand. And, I was sick and tired of being sick and tired.

In my sophomore year of high school I became very ill. Antibiotics administered monthly would not keep the sinus infections under control. Once my sinuses had to be "opened," which involved inserting a wooden stick tipped with cotton into each nostrial and pushing it up into the sinus cavities, causing excruciating pain. They were left in for 15 minutes, and relief from the procedure was short-lived.

At that time emotional problems became severe—I was extremely depressed, discouraged, and suicidal. Symptoms occurred whenever I left my home. I would experience symptoms including hot and cold flashes, fear of fainting, feeling as though I were about to faint, and extreme anxiety attacks.

Constant sinus drainage made my throat sore, and my neck was very swollen, which made me extremely nervous. The doctor recommended a tonsillectomy, which I refused until one night when my neck became so swollen that I became extremely nervous from the feeling and thought I would go crazy. I just wanted to scream. The tonsils were removed and found to be growing down into my neck, rather than out into my throat. They were two inches long. I had to take antibiotics monthly the year prior to surgery and also the year after, and I used nasal spray on a daily basis and took Actifed. Health problems weren't nearly as severe after that, although the extreme fatigue, headaches, and allergies persisted.

The following summer my mother began managing the ice cream store across the street from where we lived. That year and the next I had access to all the ice cream and toppings I wanted (and I frequently consumed as much as a quart a day), as well as ice cold slushes (half-frozen sugar water with fruit flavoring and color). At age 18, in college, I went to an allergist and had the usual tests. He found that I was allergic to many environmental factors, including various pollens, animals, fur, feathers, and dust, as well as the nasal spray that I had been using nightly for many years. I received shots twice weekly for a time, then once a week for five years. The shots helped somewhat while I received them, but they never cured me. Living on my own, my diet consisted of Oreo cookies, Cokes, Velveeta cheese sandwiches, TV dinners, cookies, hot dogs, ketchup, ice cream, chocolate, cakes, fruit, milk shakes, french fries, and cheeseburgers.

About age 21 I began eating a high protein, low carbohydrate diet, made up of cheese, fish, meat, butter, and salads, plus lots of coffee, tea, and ice cold diet pop. I was married two years later; my husband had asthma and allergies. We began going to two M.D.s who were holistically-oriented. Their allergy treatments required us to fast for 12 hours before receiving shots: five hours before that we were to expose ourselves to anything we reacted to (cats, dust, pollen, feathers, etc.). Urine specimens were then collected, centrifuged, and injected into a fleshy area in the buttocks. This series of eight treatments helped a little, but never eliminated our problems. And they were expensive.

Almost three years ago I began practicing macrobiotics and after a time my allergies improved quite remarkably. The fatigue has greatly decreased and has been replaced by an energy that allows me to be active and productive from the time I arise until bed time. Other benefits include:

—No more pimple outbreaks. My skin looks much clearer and is softer than ever before. I cut out all make-up except for mascara.

—I have not worn a deodorant for over 2 1/2 years. Previously I had to "check" constantly, since most of the time after only two or three hours my deodorant would no longer be effective.

—My hair was always dull, thin, and would split off when it reached ear lobe level, forcing me to keep it short. Now it is very thick, long, and has no split ends. It's shiny, too.

The practice of macrobiotics has brought many changes to my life: macrobiotics has altered more than just what I put on my table. Sometimes it has been very trying as I grow and change in ways that family and friends find themselves unable to understand. Yet, I would not go back to my old lifestyle for anything. An undercurrent of excitement courses through me now as I see myself changing and opening up to things around me that were always there for me to see, if I'd only been looking.

Allergies: Bill Tims, Fayetteville, Arkansas

Before I was seven years old I had many earaches and sore throats. As it was the common suggestion of doctors, I decided that removing my tonsils would eliminate the source of these problems, because they were continually becoming inflammed. (I never considered their inflammation a natural bodily defense against poisons entering my system.) Shortly after having this tonsillectomy I began to develop more and more intense allergies. Each time I had a violent sneezing attack, my parents and I decided upon some *obvious* external cause: weeds, sunflowers, cats, dust, etc. However, as time went by, it seemed as though the number of things I was allergic to was growing larger and larger, until I found myself surrounded by an alien world. My natural environment was mysterious and often evil when causing me to sneeze *without any reason at all.*

As my allergies came and left with the changing seasons, I was dealing with a much deeper sickness within myself. Sometimes conscious, sometimes unconscious, never talked about with friends, was a vacancy within myself, a lack of vitality. School did not offer solutions to this. Church did not offer solutions to this. Sometimes I felt alive with friends, only to realize when I was alone that it had been their efforts and not mine. I can remember going hunting with my father and watching his bird-dogs run all day long, up and down gulleys, across meadows and fields, disappearing and reappearing, never tiring. That hunger, that sense of search and adventure, was what I wanted to feel in my heart. Over-weight, lazy, lacking challenge and initiative, I passively assumed any role necessary for coping with various social situations.

Amidst all this there came to me a ragged copy of a book entitled the *Book of Judgment* by George Ohsawa, which introduced a way of life called macrobiotics. It made complete, stunning sense to me. In a very short time, through good friends I found out that a man named Michio Kushi had studied with Mr. Ohsawa and was teaching macrobiotics in

Boston. I came to Boston to study with him. Among other things, he told me that my overconsumption of dairy foods, sugar and liquids were the major causes of my allergies and excess weight. He suggested that I eliminate these from my diet and begin to take grains, vegetables, beans and sea vegetables as my principal foods. After two months of following his recommendations, I had lost 30 pounds and in six months my allergies were under complete control. Over the years I have begun to feel an intense aliveness within myself, surging and radiating at the roots. I find that I can share and develop understanding with friends, without our relationships being consumed in too many thoughts or emotions. To these friends, to my parents who have always tried to teach me native common sense I am grateful. I am also grateful to Mr. Ohsawa and Mr. Kushi for a glimpse at the infinite universe and its unifying principle of yin and yang, whereby I can carry on my life and my study with order and direction.

Hay Fever: Susan Stayman, Boston, Massachusetts——

Ever since Sue was twelve years old, she had hay fever every spring. She would sneeze, cough, and sniffle her way through the months of May and June—supposedly the most beautiful time of the year in New England. Those months were always a time of exams, and parties. Studying and sociability did not come easy:

"I couldn't think or look my best. I felt that my exams were always done much less well than if I had taken them in December. In fact, I did get better grades on tests taken in the winter. I took many antihistamines and found they helped quite a bit—they made me go right to sleep so I didn't feel a thing. I was like a confused bear, sleeping in spring, flunking exams and dozing stuffy-faced at parties."

Sue describes her spring allergy experience as an 8- to 10-week period of "incapacitation." While the flowers and trees came out in all their glory Sue stayed indoors, watching and waiting. There were a variety of antihistamine tablets to choose from—both prescription and non-prescription. Out of a combination of boredom and a feeling of helplessness Sue took them at random, and often thought about the coming late summer and fall when she would be free to go out and play like all the others.

Having already stopped eating meat several years before, when Sue was eighteen years old she began experimenting by eliminating dairy foods from her diet as well, only during the spring months. This practice alleviated her hay fever symptoms considerably, and gave her new hope for a less stuffy future.

It wasn't until the spring of 1981, when Sue began eating macrobiotically that she made the connection between dairy foods and sugar, particularly fruits, fruit juices, and refined sugar products. By not eating any animal food or refined sugar products, and by limiting her intake of liquid, she no longer suffers the sneezing, coughing, and dripping of hay fever.

About her recovery, Sue comments: "Hay fever doesn't kill you—at least not right away. It does indicate that the body is out of balance. By suppressing the symptoms we ignore the cause, which tends to grow into a more severe illness. . . . I'm glad to have found macrobiotics for many reasons, not the least of which is the fact that the skin around my nose is no longer made raw by the frantic, futile dabbing of tissues during the spring months of the year."

Asthma: Jon Pell, Jamaica Plain, Massachusetts

Jon Pell is a twenty-five years old restaurant owner and manager of the Five Seasons in Jamaica Plain, Massachusetts. Together with his brother Rob, Jon puts much of his time and energy into the preparation of quality natural foods. He is energetic, good-humored, and healthy—a combination of personal qualities which are becoming increasingly rare in modern times. One's first impression might be that Jon's strong vitality is the cumulative result of 25 years of sound health. In actuality, his history is quite different.

During his childhood Jon enjoyed the luxuries of Jewish upper-middle class life. His family's diet consisted primarily of animal food—mostly dairy products and meat—as well as sugar and sweet-tasting foods. In those days it was thought beneficial to eat more rich food, so red meat was thought superior to white meat, while vegetables were more a side dish. Throughout his youth, Jon was actively involved in sports, his favorites being (in order): basketball (winter), football (fall), and, lastly, baseball (spring).

At age six he was diagnosed as having asthma and other miscellaneous allergies. The family doctor began injecting possible allergens to determine the agents which elicited his allergic response. The diagnosis marked the beginning of a long and arduous odyssey with allergy. Once a week for 10 years, Jon would get "immunized" with a small dose of dandelion extract combined with minute traces of various animal by-products. After each injection and within several hours, his arm would swell up, very red and sore. These uncomfortable effects lasted at least half a day. In the spring-time the dosage was increased five-fold. Also, as there were doctors in the family, an ample supply of drugs (antihistamines: dimetap and dimetane) was always on hand. On returning from school or retiring to bed Jon took them excessively ("for comfort") on a daily basis. After two years he also began taking copious amounts of aspirin to relieve his persistent headaches. At that time he was uncertain as to whether the headaches were due to his condition or to the fact that he hated school.

Throughout the first year the treatment was very potent. Then, gradually, it began to wear off, but Jon continued to take it on faith and increased his antihistamine intake. At age 12 or 13 he began to question the efficacy of the drugs. He could "literally sneeze one hundred times at a time without pause"; huge bags had formed under his eyes and breathing was intensely difficult—sometimes "impossible." At age 14 Jon abandoned the treatment, but, very soon after, had a reaction. He decided to go back on. Then, at age 16 Jon boldly threw away all the medicine before heading off to work at a summer camp. He knew that the treatment was not working; it was time to play.

The following year Jon began eating natural foods, eliminating—for the most part—dairy products, meat, and refined sugar. The results were dramatic: within three months he was about 75 to 80 percent better. At age 18, through his brother's *shiatsu* instructor, Jon learned about macrobiotics and began eating accordingly. The recovery was soon complete; the asthmatic suffering was over.

Now a successful married father of three, Jon clearly realizes the relation between diet and his recovery:

"I was a sugar addict since a very young age. I had a box of candy hidden in my room, and also ate a lot of cheese and fruits. Back then I was really violent—I'd beat up almost anyone. So, although I knew all along I was okay, I visited a psychiatrist throughout my teen years until I found natural foods.

"The dairy products were the root of the problem. Before and after beginning the natural foods I could eat tons of sugar and never have a reaction. Then I'd add dairy and my lungs would soon fill with mucus; the attacks came with deadly consistency. To sum it all up: the word cheese rhymes with the words sneeze and wheeze, and it creates all of those."

Nowadays Jon radiates with stamina and clarity. His appreciation for macrobiotics is reflected in his highly energetic approach to cooking and in his bright outlook on life. Springtime is no longer a season to fear.

Hay Fever, Food Allergies, Miscellaneous Allergies: Susan C. Segal, Brookline, Massachusetts

As a child, Susan loved both ice cream and whipped cream. For the first 25 years of her life she claims that these were her "staple"—consuming them three or four times each week in her teenage years. Curiously enough she did not like milk very much, and never touched sour cream, cream cheese or mayonnaise. During college, however, she was a cheese gourmet, and consumed large quantities of the harder cheeses for all four years. During this time Susan gained a lot of weight, most of which became concentrated in her thighs and hips.

Susan's allergies began in early childhood, with the primary culprits being two foods—eggs and chocolate. These would induce intense sneezing as she ate them. The allergies were actually multiple, including a heavy case of hay fever during the spring and summer months. One other allergen was cigarette smoke, which would cause all of the symptoms of hay fever as well as congested bronchi and wheezing. Also in the two years of college she discovered that she was allergic to penicillin. It would cause various areas of her face to swell.

Treatments involved all kinds of medication, primarily non-prescription. These included Contac, Ilosone, Actifed, Bendryl (a depressant), and special bronchi dilating liquids such as cough syrups. The drugs never seemed to do the job completely, and Susan was constantly looking for something better.

In October of 1980, at age 26, Susan began the macrobiotic diet after discovering a golf-ball size tumor at the left-side base of the skull. At this time she was also experiencing large mood swings as well as reproductive problems. Her macrobiotic counselor advised a very simple diet of whole grains, soups, beans, and land and sea vegetables, for four months. Very soon after beginning this regimen, all of her allergic symptoms began to disappear. The following spring Susan noticed that her hay fever was gone. While the tumor still exists and is gradually diminishing, Susan is grateful for the relief of her allergic condition. Of course, she no longer eats eggs and chocolate; but as she says, "Who needs them anyway?"

Allergies: Edward Esko, Brookline, Massachusetts

I would like to relate my personal experience with macrobiotic healing. Throughout my childhood and adolescence, I suffered from what were diagnosed as "allergies." This meant that practically every day of my life I would sneeze repeatedly and my nose would often run. This was a year-round problem, and became even worse with the coming of late-summer and "hay-fever" season, when I would experience minor swelling in my nasal cavity and around my eyes.

Periodically, this chronic condition would erupt into a full-scale infection which included fever, mucus in my chest and bronchi region, and general bodily weakness, for which regular doses of penicillin and antibiotics were usually prescribed. Once, when I was eight years old, this infection appeared in my throat and was diagnosed as "tonsillitis," after which my tonsils and adenoid glands were removed.

In the meantime, this chronic condition continued, during which it was inconceivable for me to go anywhere without a package of tissues, or to go to sleep without a box of tissues next to my bed. Because of this it was difficult to concentrate on my work at school or to fully participate and enjoy life. From time to time, my parents would become concerned and attempt to discover the substance or substances that I was "allergic to." The new rug in the house, the horse-hair in the mattress, the feathers in the pillow, and, of course, the mysterious and obscure "pollen," were all considered as possibly being responsible. At one point, I went to an "allergy specialist," who proceeded to inject the inner part of my forearm with about 15 different substances in an attempt to identify the culprit. Tiny lumps and red spots developed where practically all the needles were inserted, and, according to the doctor, the results were "inconclusive." The mystery continued.

Occasionally I would have strange reactions to animals, particularly cats. At times, if I would come in contact with an ordinary house-cat, I would sneeze repeatedly and my eyes would water, and if I touched the cat, my skin would often break out into red spots that itched.

At the age of 20, I dscovered the philosophy of Oriental medicine, which, when applied to the selection and preparation of daily food, is called macrobiotics. According to this philosophy, my condition was a result of the quality of my blood, which was determined by what I had been eating—particularly foods such as milk and milk products, sugar, animal fats, fruits, and excess liquid—and not by external factors such as pollen, chicken feathers, horse hair, and so on.

Interestingly enough, when I began to eat whole grains, beans, cooked fresh vegetables, sea vegetables, *miso*, and other wholesome foods, and eliminated ice cream, candy, milk, cheese, butter, meat, etc., from my diet, the symptoms I had experienced all my life disappeared one by one. As an example, the friends with whom I was living had several cats as pets. At first, it was difficult to be in the same room with them without sneezing, my eyes watering, or my skin breaking out. Because of my condition, I was unable to live in harmony with ordinary house-cats, or to have them as my friends. However, after eating macrobiotically for only two days, all of these symptoms disappeared. In fact, on the second evening of the new diet, one of the cats slept on my bed. I suffered none of the previous symptoms, and had gained a new friend.

Also, I am no longer troubled by sneezing, runny-nose, and watery eyes, and no longer carry tissues or a handkerchief, and have not taken any form of medication for the last five years. The mystery was at long last solved. I have experienced many other benefits as a result of macrobiotics, and I hope to relate them at some future time. In the meantime, I hope my story will be of benefit to others who have experienced similar difficulties. Thank you.

Annotated Medical References

Anderson, L. *et al.* (1970); "Melon and banana sensitivity coincident with ragweed pollinosis"; *J. Allerg.* 45: 310

The synergistic influence of eating tropical fruits (as well as vegetables of tropical origin) is a mysterious "coincidence" for modern medicine. Hay fever sufferers were found to exhibit greater oral pruritis (throat and mouth itchiness) after eating cantaloupe, banana, honeydew melon or watermelon.

Bahna, S. L., Heiner, D. C. (1980); *Allergies to Milk;* Grune & Stration, N.Y.

Tropical fruits appear to reinforce allergic reactivity. page 155. In one study, lactose intolerance occurred in more than 50% of patients with severe gastrointestinal milk allergy. page 111.

Bierman, C., Pierson, W., and Donaldson, J. (1970); "The evaluation of middle ear function in children"; *Am. J. Dis. Child.* 120: 233

A variety of complications are associated with asthma and hay fever, including nose, throat, and ear problems. While the stuffy nose is the better-known symptom, also quite common are ear infections, ear pain, and ear popping or plugging, and hearing difficulties. Severe ear problems can impair a child's speech development, and also give the impression of being "dumb," inattentive or not alert. This often leads to a poor rapport with the child's teacher as well as social alienation. Ear problems are a result of the expansion or swelling of the lower end of the eustachian tubes. Out of 1,222 allergic infants, 23% had evidence of abnormal ear function.

Bier, O. G., Dias da Silva, W., Gotze, D., Mota, I. (1981); *Fundamentals of Immunology;* Springer-Verlag, N.Y., N.Y. 442 pages.

The complementary-antagonistic relationship between B-cells and T-cells was gleaned from this book: spiral configurations in spleen, p. 27/memory, p. 36/microvilli length, p. 50/cell density, p. 51/lifespan, p. 366/Other characteristics were also obtained from this book, as well as from a college Immunology course.

Biering-Sorensen, F., Jorgensen, T., Hilden, J. (1978); "Sudden infant death in Copenhagen 1956–1971. I. Infant feeding." *Acta Pediatr. Scand.* 67: 129–137.

Sudden infant death syndrome (SIDS) has been linked with cow's milk allergy. Researchers hypothesize that formula-fed infants given cow's milk shortly before sleeping regurgitate some stomach contents and aspirate a small amount of the milk into the lungs, where it triggers an acute allergic reaction and sudden death. This hypothesis arose from a number of studies which noted that bottle-fed infants more commonly develop SIDS than breast-fed infants.

Bleumink, E., Young, E. (1968); "Identification of the atopic allergen in cow's milk"; *Int. Arch. Allergy.* 34: 521–543.

Neither milk fat nor lactose itself has been found to be antigenic. It seems, however, that the allergenicity of cow's milk protein is enhanced (a synergistic effect) by reacting with lactose. In milk-hypersensitive individuals, the skin reactivity to beta-lactoglobulin (milk protein) was increased a hundredfold by prior reacting of the protein with lactose.

Bricklin, A. S., (1976); "Natural healing, the ultimate: how the body defends and repairs itself"; in: *The Practical Encyclopedia of Natural Healing;* Bricklin, M. (ed), Rodale Press, Inc., Emmaus, Pa. pp. 179–185; 332–359.

Exercise is beneficial to allergic people. Physical activity produces a constricting effect (yang) in the small blood vessels and symptoms improve in a matter of three to five minutes. Aerobic exercises, swimming, bicycling and vigorous yoga are all appropriate. page 181.

Bullen, C. L., Tearle, P. V., Stewart, M. G. (1977); "The effect of "humanised" milks and supplemented breast feeding on the faecal flora of infants"; *J. Med. Microbiol.* 10: 403–13.

The use of formula milks as well as supplementation of vitamins and mineral pills by the mother increases the infant's susceptibility to allergy. Ingestion of cow's milk formulas upsets the natural balance of intestinal bacteria and introduces many toxigenic flora, thereby apparently predisposing the infant to allergic tendencies. By taking excessive amounts of supplements while breastfeeding, the mother may weaken her child's immune system. At the present time, the only reliable system of moderate supplementation (necessary only when an individual is unable to obtain essential nutrients—such as vitamin B_{12}—directly from the food) is the clinical kinesiology approach.

Davidson, J. (1981); "When allergies cause mental illness"; *Chimo:* July/August pp. 18–23.

In cerebral food allergies, the antigen-antibody response causes the blood vessels and membranes of the brain to swell, and this probably induces changes in mood.

Mood and behavioral changes include: lack of energy and ambition, drowsiness, depression, inability to think and concentrate, temper tantrums and emotional instability. (Note: these all suggest a weak intestinal condition.)

Eastham, E., and Walker, W. (1977); "Effect of cow's milk on the GI tract: a persistent dilemma for the pediatrician"; *Pedia.* 60: 477.

Human milk contains a factor, called IgA, which stimulates development of the intestinal mucosa. Furthermore, IgA antibodies can prevent the transport of foreign or potentially allergenic protein molecules across the gut wall. Mother's milk provides much IgA, and is therefore deemed helpful in the prevention of cow's milk and other food allergies. (By contrast, cow's milk provides primarily IgG, which appears to have an addititive effect on the allergic IgE response.) However, it should be emphasized that while mother's milk contains many essential natural resistance factors, its entire quality is dependent on mother's diet. Harmful antigens introduced by mother's diet can still penetrate the infant's relatively leaky gut via the mother's breast milk. Subsequent studies have revealed that some degree of IgA deficiency precedes the majority of infantile allergic disorders.

Eaton, K. K. (1982); "The incidence of allergy—has it changed?"; *Clin. Allergy* 12: 107–110.

A survey of the entire population of a new-town general practice, comparing the years 1974 with 1979, showed an overall statistically significant rise in the incidence of allergies for both sexes. Hay fever and asthma continued to show a male dominance.

Galton, L. (1977); "Allergies"; in: *Medical Advances*, Crown Publishers, Inc. N.Y. pp 4–12.

Wheat is the most allergenic of the small grains, while rye is the least allergenic. page 12.

Glaser, J. and Johnstone, D. (1953); "Prophylaxis of allergic disease in children"; *JAMA* 153: 620.

With a milk-, egg-, and wheat-free diet, infants during the first nine months of life showed a marked decrease in the incidence of atopic eczema. Also, of those who did develop eczema, only 15% subsequently developed asthma or hay fever compared to 60% of their eczematous siblings on the control diet (with dairy).

Grulee, C. G., Sanford, H. N., Herron, P. H. (1934); "Breast and artificial feeding"; *JAMA* 103: 734.

20,061 babies were studied for at least nine months in the Infant Welfare Society. Gastrointestinal (GI) and respiratory infections were significantly more frequent ($p<0.001$) in infants not fed breast milk. Specifically, deaths from GI infections were sixteen-fold and from respiratory infections over 120-fold more common in cow's-milk-fed than breast-fed infants.

Grulee, C. G., Sanford, N. H. (1936); "The influence of breast feeding on infantile eczema"; *J. Pediatr.* 9: 223.

The authors report a greater than sevenfold increase in infantile atopic eczema in non-breast-milk-fed babies, suggesting that feeding cow's milk to infants promóted the manifestation of allergic tendencies.

Hamburger, R. N. (1979); "Allergy Research"; *Yearbook of Science and the Future*, Encyclopedia Britannica, Inc. Chicago, pp. 367–370.

The author states the following: "A recently completed study confirmed that environmental controls such as strict breast feeding and reduced intake of cow's milk by the mother, and diet and living areas with low tendencies to induce allergic reactions did indeed result in a lower incidence of allergic symptoms in a baby during the first two years of life. They did not, however, significantly lower the baby's serum IgE levels (genetically determined) compared with those of the control group." page 368–9.
* This study points to the possibility that the quantity of IgE is not as important as the quality of these components.

Hamburger, R. N. (1978); "Of many things"; *Ann. Allergy*. 40: 374.

The total number of lymphocytes (lymph cells) in the human body is about 2,000,000,000,000 (two billion), with one billion T-cells and one billion B-cells. About one million new lymphocytes are formed in the body each second! A single plasma cell (which is differentiated from a B-cell), can synthesize and pump into the blood some 2,000 antibodies per second! What incredibly dynamic balance the immune system is able to maintain.

Harfouche, J. K. (1970); "The importance of breast-feeding"; *J. Trop. Pediatr.* 16: 133–175.

Tropical fruits and vegetables such as tomatoes, rhubarb, spinach, spices, and garlic have a potentiating effect on allergic reactivity.

Jackson, A. A., Golden, M. H. N. (1978); "The Human Rumen"; *Lancet*. October, 7, 1978. pp. 764–766.

"Children who are fed a calf's diet tend to develop a rumen." This leads to chronic diarrea and malnutrition, accompanied by the multiple generation of toxin-producing bacteria in the upper small intestine. These effects may account for symptoms ascribed to cow's-milk-protein allergy.

Jacobson, M. F. (1976); *Eater's Digest, The Consumer's Factbook of Food Additives;* Anchor Books.

"Today's foods contain more than $485,000,000 worth of several thousand food additives." p. 4.

Jensen, D. (1980); *The Principles of Physiology;* 2nd edition. Appleton-Century-Crofts, N.Y., N.Y.

Stem cells are converted to B-cells in several tissues, including the appendix and other intestinal lymphoid tissues, liver and spleen. p. 527.

Minor, R. *et al.* (1974); "Greater frequency of viral respiratory infections in asthmatic children as compared with nonasthmatic sibs"; *J. Pediatr.* 85: 472.

Acute viral respiratory infections in infants and children frequently occur with or precede asthma attacks.

Morrison-Smith, J. (1973); "Skin tests and atopic allergy in children"; *Clin. Allergy.* 3: 269.

The researchers found a lower incidence of asthma in children of African origin who were born outside Britain. (Note: one of the primary differences between the British and the African diet is the former's heavy inclusion of white sugar, as well as more dairy and animal foods overall.) More importantly, offspring of parents of African origin who were born in Britain had at least as high an incidence of allergy as indigenous non-African children. This confirms that the difference in incidence of asthma in African children was an environmental one rather than genetic.

National Center for Health Statistics, U.S. Dept. of Health, Education and Welfare. Public Health Service Publication. No. 2121, Rockville, Md.

There are significantly higher incidences of asthma in boys than in girls.

Ogle, K. A., Bullock, J. D. (1980); "Children with allergic rhinitis and/or bronchial asthma treated with elimination diet: a five-year follow-up"; *Ann. Allergy.* 44: 86.

322 children under one year of age with respiratory and skin allergies were placed on a 6 week "hypoallergenic diet," which excluded milk, egg, chocolate, soy, and cereals. The diet consisted of beef, carrots, broccoli, and apricots. Upon subsequent introduction, milk and eggs were shown to be most allergenic and cereal grains were least allergenic. Most but not all children reacted upon allergen "challenge." Furthermore, five years later, only 6% of the group showed any evidence of food allergy, while a large percentage (40%) had respiratory allergy. Thus most children apparently "outgrow" food allergy and "grow into" inhalant/respiratory allergy.

Rapaport, H. G., Linde, S. M. (1970); *The Complete Allergy Guide;* Simon & Schuster, N.Y., N.Y.

At least half of the entire world may suffer from one or anther form of allergy. (p. 13)
100 million Americans are estimated to have allergies. (p. 14)

1/3 of all children under 17 yrs. old with chronic diseases are estimated to have allergies. (p. 14)

Concerning biological rhythms in allergic reactivity: Atopic asthma occurs most frequently between 11 p.m. and 4 a.m.. This is the time when adrenal

Juto, P. (1980); "Elevated immunoglobulin E in T-cell deficient infants fed cow's milk"; *J. Allerg. & Clin. Immunol.* 66: 402.

A high proportion of infants allergic to cow's milk also had a lower number of T-cells. Furthermore, babies fed cow's milk developed more allergy symptoms than breast fed babies. The resulting allergies were not necessarily due to cow's-milk-protein hypersensitivity.

Kaufman, H. and Frick, O. (1979); "Incidence of asthma in bottle-fed infants"; Presented at the Annual Congress of the American College of Allergists, San Francisco, Ca. January, 1979.

Babies who were breast-fed for six weeks were considerably less likely to develop asthma or infantile atopic dermatitis than those given cow's milk formulae. Ninety-four full-term infants of ninety-two mothers were followed prospectively for two years. Only two of 38 breast-fed infants developed asthma, while 10 of 56 cow's-milk-fed infants developed became asthmatic during the study. (Speculation: if the nursing mother had avoided dairy products altogether there would have been a complete absence of asthma in this group, since mother's milk is ultimately transmuted from her daily diet. Unfortunately, no such studies exist to substantiate this conjecture.) In sum, major allergic disease during the first two years of life can be largely prevented by the practice of breast-feeding.

Light, W. and Wartley, G. (1980); "Effect of maternal asthma on newborn"; *J. Allerg. & Clin. Immunol.* 65: 204.

A history of maternal asthma, symptomatic during pregnancy, is associated with an increased incidence of respiratory distress and/or jaundice in the newborn. In other words, the mother's respiratory weaknesses are conferred on the newborn, manifesting in both respiratory and digestive/metabolic/immune (liver-related) weaknesses. In Oriental medicine, the respiratory and digestive systems have a complementary and antagonistic relationship. The constitution of these systems is passed on by the mother, whereas the constitution of the nervous system is acquired primarily from the father.

Mariano, F. L. V., Hill, R. B. (1975); "Immunologic injury"; in: *Principles of Pathobiology*, 2nd edition; Oxford University Press, N.Y., N.Y. pp. 173–201.

Scientists have observed that the allergic antibodies (IgE) have an unusual affinity for skin and mucous membranes, and tend to become fixed to basophils and mast cells. These "reagins" have consequently been designated as an "abnormal class" of antibodies. Japanese scientists have determined that these abnormal antibodies result from the splitting of normal antibodies (a yin process) in such a way as to produce a cell-fixing antibody. (p. 186)

Allergic disorders are restricted almost entirely to man. (p. 187) (Humans have probably played a hand in those seen in animals, however, by instigating artificial or abnormal eating patterns and environmental pollutants.)

"Not all individuals exposed to antigen develop hypersensitivity. On the other hand, most individuals who are allergic to one antigen are allergic to several antigens. Frequently several members of the same family are atopic. Thus, predisposition to atopic hypersensitivity is thought by some to be hereditary; but the evidence supporting this suggestion is circumstantial, and no known genetic mechanism is compatible with the existing data." (p. 187)

Luoma, R., Koivikko, A. (1982); "Occurrence of atopic disease in three generations;" *Scand. J. Soc. Med.* 10: 49–56.

Potentially allergic children cannot be adequately selected (predicted) on the basis of the family history of allergic disease. In this study, only 46% of atopic children had an atopic parent.

Luoma, R. Koivikko, A., Viander, M. (1983); "Development of asthma, allergic rhinitis, and atopic dermatitis by the age of five years"; *Allergy.* 38: 339–346.

A number of studies have found *normal* IgE levels in atopic disease. These studies of allergic individuals have failed to demonstrate a significant difference between the normal range of serum IgE and the serum IgE levels presumably associated with allergic disorders.

Matthew, D. *et al.* (1977); "Prevention of Eczema"; *Lancet.* 1: 321.

In perhaps one of the most respectable studies to date, the researchers conducted a program of strict breast-feeding, delay in immunizations, and avoidance of pets in the home. They reported a significant lowering of atopic eczema and asthma in newborns.

Michel, F. *et al.* (1980); "Comparison of clinical and immunologic parameters for the prediction of infant allergy"; (abstract) *J. Allergy. Clin. Immunol.* 65: 167.

The fact of embryonic education via the mother's diet and physiological condition is suggested by the following observation: allergic tendencies in the mother are a more important factor in the child's susceptibility than allergic tendencies in the father. The father's biological influence (passed on by sperm) appears to be negligible. This study found that allergic sensitization of the fetus to cow's milk can take place *in utero* (in the womb), even though the mother herself may have *no* milk hypersensitivity. Therefore, whether the mother was allergic to milk or not, her dairy consumption and imbalanced eating practices produced allergic tendencies in the newborn. The scientists suggest that mothers should seriously consider limiting their consumption of dairy and other "allergenic" foods during pregnancy.

Minor, R. *et al.* (1974); "Greater frequency of viral respiratory infections in asthmatic children as compared with nonasthmatic sibs"; *J. Pediatr.* 85: 472.

Acute viral respiratory infections in infants and children frequently occur with or precede asthma attacks.

Morrison-Smith, J. (1973); "Skin tests and atopic allergy in children"; *Clin. Allergy.* 3: 269.

The researchers found a lower incidence of asthma in children of African origin who were born outside Britain. (Note: one of the primary differences between the British and the African diet is the former's heavy inclusion of white sugar, as well as more dairy and animal foods overall.) More importantly, offspring of parents of African origin who were born in Britain had at least as high an incidence of allergy as indigenous non-African children. This confirms that the difference in incidence of asthma in African children was an environmental one rather than genetic.

National Center for Health Statistics, U.S. Dept. of Health, Education and Welfare. Public Health Service Publication. No. 2121, Rockville, Md.

There are significantly higher incidences of asthma in boys than in girls.

Ogle, K. A., Bullock, J. D. (1980); "Children with allergic rhinitis and/or bronchial asthma treated with elimination diet: a five-year follow-up"; *Ann. Allergy.* 44: 86.

322 children under one year of age with respiratory and skin allergies were placed on a 6 week "hypoallergenic diet," which excluded milk, egg, chocolate, soy, and cereals. The diet consisted of beef, carrots, broccoli, and apricots. Upon subsequent introduction, milk and eggs were shown to be most allergenic and cereal grains were least allergenic. Most but not all children reacted upon allergen "challenge." Furthermore, five years later, only 6% of the group showed any evidence of food allergy, while a large percentage (40%) had respiratory allergy. Thus most children apparently "outgrow" food allergy and "grow into" inhalant/respiratory allergy.

Rapaport, H. G., Linde, S. M. (1970); *The Complete Allergy Guide;* Simon & Schuster, N.Y., N.Y.

At least half of the entire world may suffer from one or anther form of allergy. (p. 13)
100 million Americans are estimated to have allergies. (p. 14)

1/3 of all chronic diseases in children under 17 yrs. old are estimated to have allergies. (p. 14)

Concerning biological rhythms in allergic reactivity: Atopic asthma occurs most frequently between 11 p.m. and 4 a.m.. This is the time when adrenal hormone production is lowest. Also, when blood pressure, lung function, and hormone secretion are lower (all yin symptoms), allergic reactivity is greatest. (p. 23)

In one study of childhood allergies, certain problematic allergens were determined in order of percentages: citrus fruits (41%); soybeans, peanuts, and peas (30%); eggs (28%); and chocolate (27%). Note that this adds up to more than 100% since most infants had more than one allergy. Cow's milk is the number one allergen. (p. 30)

Roberts, S. A., Soothill, J. F. (1982); "Provocation of allergic response by supplementary feeds of cow's milk"; *Arch. Dis. Child.* 57: 127–130.

Although this study involved rats instead of humans, it is highly important. When cow's milk was fed to rats in early life, there was a subsequent *increase* in allergic tendencies in later life. These later allergies were not related to cow's milk antigen. Human studies may require a longer time period to confirm this effect. This is one of the first studies to clearly suggest that feeding cows' milk might predispose to allergy in an antigen non-specific way. With regard to the influence of dairy food on allergy, this study marks a shift from the secondary viewpoint of "sensitivity" to the primary issue of "susceptibility."

Salk, L. *et al.*, (1974); "Perinatal complications in the history of asthmatic children"; *Am. J. Dis. Child.* 127: 30.

Birth complications appear to significantly increase the child's chances of developing asthma. In a retrospective study, randomly selected asthmatic children born on the same day in the same obstetrical unit were compared to either of two control groups. There was a significantly greater number of asthmatic children who had had two or three neonatal complications for mother and/or child compared to either of the two control groups.

Schmidt, *et al.* (1981); "Clinical ecological study of chronic juvenile offenders"; *Int. J. Biosocial Rsh.* 2: 15–20.

A two year clinical study of 22 chronic juvenile offenders, ages 12–17, found that 90% suffered from some degrees of *food and/or environmental allergies.* Eighty-eight percent had abnormal glucose tolerance. Foods most frequently consumed included milk, white bread, refined sugar, soda, cheese, margarine, ketchup, butter, coffee, and cold cereal, though milk, white bread, and beef were by far the most prominent. Milk was consumed in excessive amounts by most offenders (5–10 eight oz glasses per day). Removal of all dairy products and refined sugar from the diet lead to reduced sinus stuffiness, improved skin condition, increased energy levels, and reduced behavioral imbalances (i.e., hostility, aggressiveness, irritability, and depression).

Smolensky, Ph.D., Reinberg M.D., Ph.D., Queng, M.D. (1981); "The chronobiology and chronopharmacology of allergy"; *Ann. Allergy.* 47: 234–252.

Several studies show that both asthma and hay fever symptoms occur more frequently in the evening and early morning hours than at other times.

Soothill, J., *et al.* (1976); "Predisposing factors and the development of reaginic allergy in infancy"; *Clin. Allergy.* 6: 305.

In Europe, asthma occurs more frequently in children born in late autumn/early winter.

Takishima, *et al.* (1932); "The bronchodilatory effect of acupuncture in patients with acute asthma"; *Ann. Allergy.* 48: 44.

The effectiveness of acupuncture therapy for asthmatic patients was studied by continuous monitoring of the respiratory function. The researchers estimated the charge of total respiratory resistance (Rrs) of asthmatic patients during their treatment by acupuncture therapy. They performed a single-blind study consisting of a placebo acupuncture, a placebo stimulation, and real acupuncture therapy. For further control of this study, they selected an easily locatable point for needle placement among the many traditional meridian points. In 10 out of 26 acupuncture therapies, Rrs significantly decreased while in only one of 17 placebo treatments did Rrs decrease. General improvement was noted overall.

Varonier, H., Hahn, W. (1966); "Cardiac and vascular reaction in atopic and nonatopic children"; *J. Allerg.* 38: 352.

Allergic individuals exhibit some peculiar autonomic nervous system responses. For example, they have higher mean heart rate and skin temperature. These studies suggest a mixed pattern of sympathetic and parasympathetic dominance, resulting in abnormal cardiac and vascular reactivity in allergic people.

Wittig, H. J., McLaughlin, E. T., Leifer, K. L., Belloit. (1978); "Risk factors for the development of allergic disease: analysis of 2,190 patient records"; *Ann. Allergy.* 41: 84–88.

Records of 2,190 patients allergic patients (including 1,143 with asthma and 557 with allergic rhinitis) were analyzed for the impact of certain risk factors on age of onset of allergic disease and on sensitization to certain antigens. Risk factors included race, sex, maternal age, family structure, life style, feeding history, environmental factors and heredity. Age of onset was significantly earlier in males, blacks, bottle-fed babies (as opposed to breast-fed), children of younger mothers, children of rural origin, children of smoking parents and children with a bilateral family history of allergy.

Resources

Further information on the macrobiotic approach to health can be obtained from the **East West Foundation,** a non-profit organization established in 1972. The East West Foundation, together with its six major affiliates or branch offices in the United States, offers ongoing public classes in macrobiotics and macrobiotic cooking, and provides private dietary and way of life counseling for those interested in individual guidance. There are also **Macrobiotics International** and **East West Centers** in Canada, Mexico, Latin America, Europe, the Middle East, Africa, Asia and Australia. The whole foods and naturally processed items described in this book and in its companion volume (*Allergies*, the Macrobiotic Food and Cooking Series) are available at thousands of natural foods and health foods stores and at growing numbers of supermarkets. The macrobiotic specialty items are also available by mail order from various distributors and retailers. An annually updated list of qualified and affiliated macrobiotic counselors and instructors is also available from the **Kushi Institute** in Boston and its affiliates in London, Amsterdam and Antwerp; the Kushi Institute is an educational institution founded in 1979 for the purpose of providing more extensive instruction on a full-time or part-time basis for those interested in becoming macrobiotic counselors and instructors.

BOSTON HEADQUARTERS
Macrotiotics International and the **East West Foundation**
17 Station Street
P.O. Box 850
Brookline, Massachusetts, 02147
(617) 738–0045

Baltimore
4803 Yellowwood Road
Baltimore, MD 21209
(301) 367–6655

Connecticut
184 East Main Street
Middletown, CT 06457
(203) 344–0090

Philadelphia
606 South Ninth Street
Philadelphia, PA 19147
(215) 922–4567

California
708 North Orange Grove Avenue
Hollywood, CA 90046
(213 651–5491

Illinois
1574 Asbury Avenue
Evanston, IL 60201
(312) 328–6632

Washington, D.C.
Box 40012
Washington, DC 20016
(301) 897–8352

The Kushi Institute
Box 1100
Brookline, Massachusetts 02147
(617) 731–0564

Bibliography

Aihara, Cornelia, *The Do of Cooking*, Oroville, Calif.; George Ohsawa Macrobiotic Foundation, 1972.

—— *Macrobiotic Kitchen: Key to Good Health*, Tokyo; Japan Publcations, 1982

Aihara, Herman, *Acid and Alkaline*, Oroville, Calif.; George Ohsawa Macrobiotic Foundation, 1980.

Ballantine, Rudolph, M.D., *Diet and Nutrition, A Holistic Approach*, Honesdale, Penn.; The Himalayan Institute, 1978.

Bieler, H. *Food is Your Best Medicine*, New York, NY; Vintage Books, 1965.

Bricklin, A. S., "Natural Healing, The Ultimate: How the Body Defends and Repairs Itself"; in *The Practical Encyclopedia of Natural Healing*, Bricklin, M. (ed.), pp. 179–185, 332–359, Emmaus, PA; Rodale Press, 1976.

Dietary Goals for the United States, Washington, D.C.,; Select Committee on Nutrition and Human Needs, U.S. Senate, 1977.

Diet, Nutrition and Cancer, Washington, D.C.; National Academy of Sciences, 1982.

Dubos, Rene, *Mirage of Health*, New York; Harper & Row, 1979.

Dufty, William, *Sugar Blues*, New York; Warner, 1975.

Esko, Edward and Wendy, *Macrobiotic Cooking for Everyone*, Tokyo; Japan Publications, 1980.

Esko, Wendy, *Introducing Macrobiotic Cooking*, Tokyo; Japan Publications, 1978.

Giannini, AV, Sculz, N.D., Chang, T.T., Wong, D.C., *The Best Guide to Allergies*, New York; Appleton-Century-Crofts, 1981.

Healthy People: The Surgeon General's Report on Health Promotion and Disease Prevention, Washington, D.C.; Government Printing Office, 1979.

Jacobsen, Michael, *The Changing American Diet*, Washington, D.C.; Center for Science in the Public Interest, 1978.

Kohler, Jean and Mary Alice, *Healing Miracles from Macrobiotics*, West Nyack, N.Y.; Parker, 1979.

Kushi, Aveline, *How to Cook with Miso*, Tokyo; Japan Publications, 1978.

Kushi, Aveline and Esko, Wendy, *The Changing Seasons Macrobiotic Cookbook*, Wayne, N.J.; Avery Publishing Group, 1984.

Kushi, Michio, *Diabetes and Hypoglycemia*, Tokyo; Japan Publications, 1985.

—— *The Book of Do-In: Exercise for Physical and Spiritual Development*, Tokyo; Japan Publications, 1979.

—— *The Book of Macrobiotics*, Tokyo; Japan Publications, 1977.

—— *Cancer and Heart Disease: The Macrobiotic Approach to Degenerative Disorders*, (Rev. ed.) Tokyo; Japan Publications, 1985.

—— *The Era of Humanity*, Brookline, Mass.; East West Journal, 1980.

—— *How to See Your Health: The Book of Oriental Diagnosis*, Tokyo; Japan Publications, 1980.

—— *The Macrobiotic Approach to Cancer*, Wayne, N.J.; Avery Publishing Group, 1982.

—— *Natural Healing Through Macrobiotic*, Tokyo; Japan Publications, 1978.

—— *Your Face Never Lies*, Wayne, N.J.; Avery Publishing Group, 1983.

Kushi, Michio and Kushi, Aveline, *Macrobiotic Pregnancy and Care of the Newborn*, Tokyo; Japan Publications, 1984.

Kushi, Michio and Jack, Alex, *The Cancer Prevention Diet*, New York; St. Martins Press, 1983.

Kushi, Michio and Jack, Alex, *Diet for A Strong Heart*, New York; St. Martins Press, 1984.

Mendelsohn, Robert, S., M.D., *Confessions of A Medical Heretic*, Chicago, Ill.; Contemporary Books, 1979.

—— *Male Practice*, Chicago, Ill.; Contemporary Books, 1980.

Miller, Saul, M.D., *Food For Thought*, Englewood Cliffs, N.J.; Prentice-Hall, 1979.

Ohsawa, George, *Cancer and the Philosophy of the Far East*, Oroville, Calif.; George Ohsawa Macrobiotic Foundation, 1971 edition.

—— *You Are All Sanpaku*, edited by William Dufty, New York University Books, 1965.

—— *Zen Macrobiotics*, Los Angeles; Ohsawa Foundation, 1965.

Ohsawa, Lima, *Macrobiotic Cuisine*, Tokyo; Japan Publications. 1984.

Sattilaro, Anthony, M.D., with Tom Monte, *Recalled By Life: The Story of My Recovery From Cancer*, Boston; Houghton-Mifflin, 1982.

Yamamoto, Shizuko, *Barefoot Shiatsu*, Tokyo; Japan Publications, 1979.

Periodicals

East West Journal, Brookline, Mass.

MacroMuse, Washington, D.C.

Nutrition Action, Washington, D.C.

"The People's Doctor" by Robert Mendelsohn, M.D. and Marian Thompson, Evanston, Ill.

Index